Y0-ALM-021

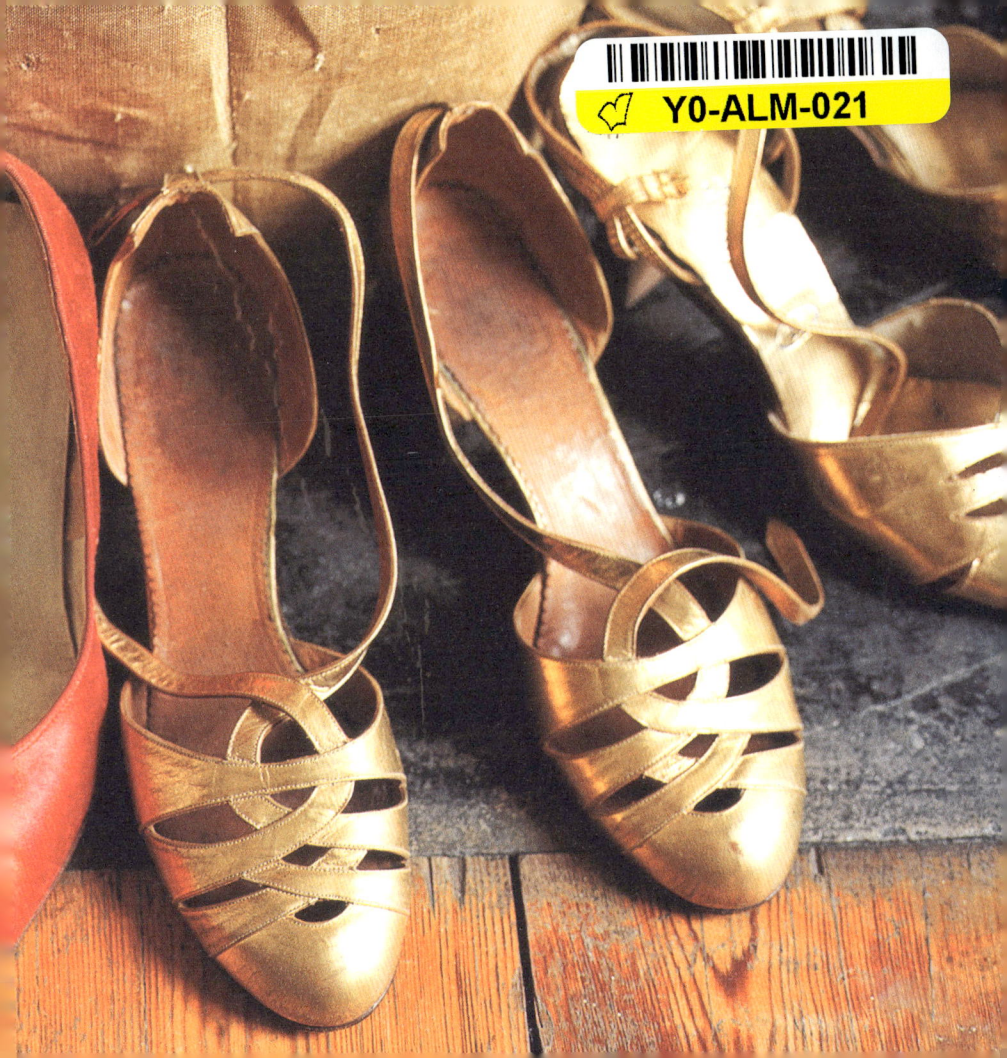

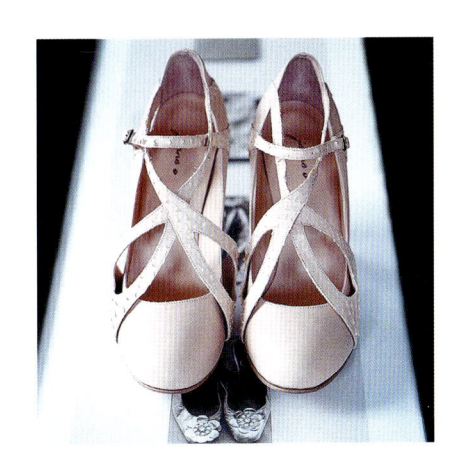

A PASSION FOR
STILETTOS

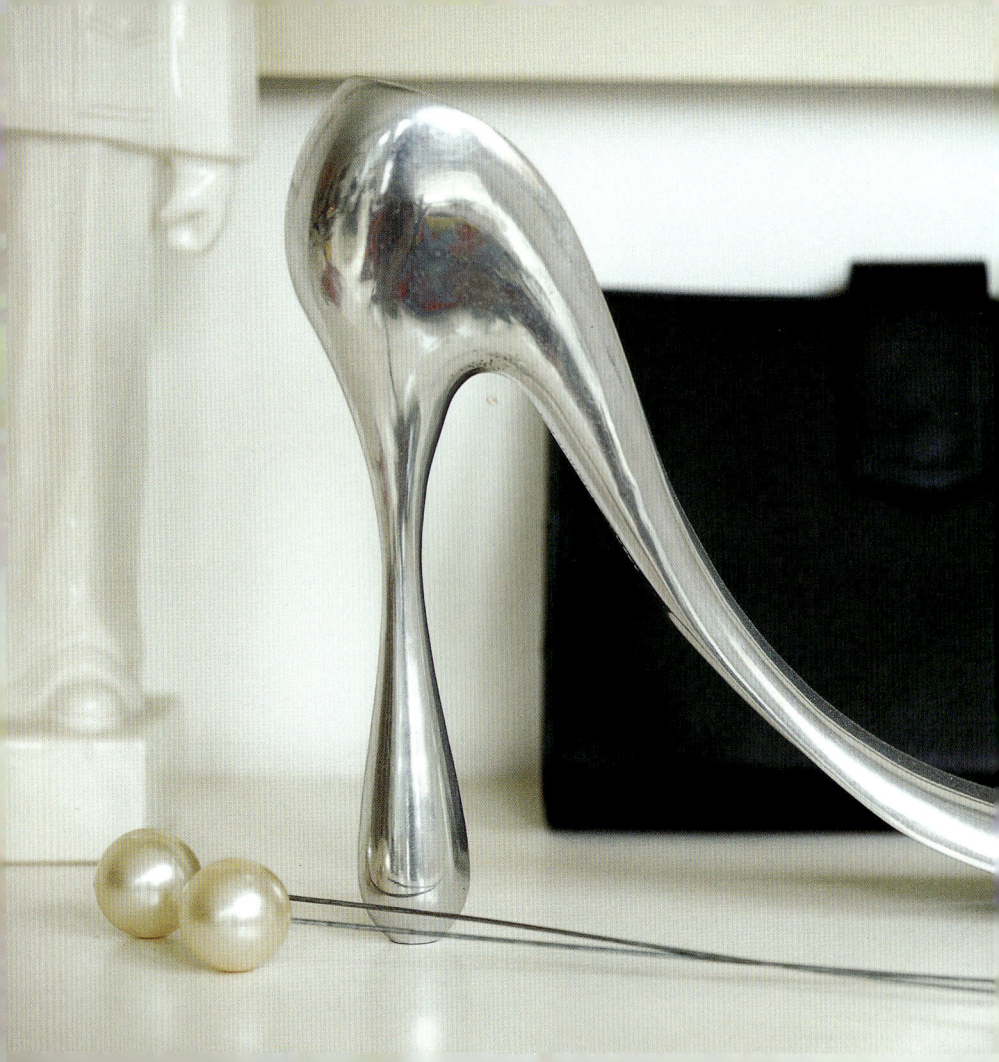

A PASSION FOR STILETTOS

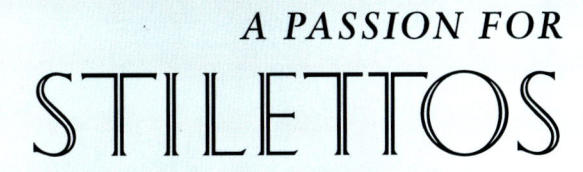

Sandra Deeble
photography by **Sandra Lane**

RYLAND
PETERS
& SMALL
LONDON NEW YORK

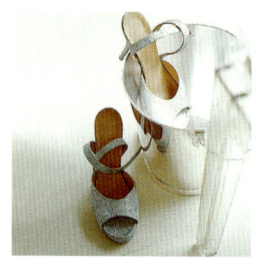

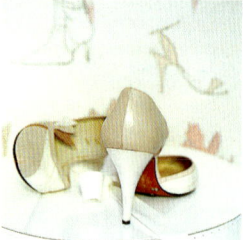

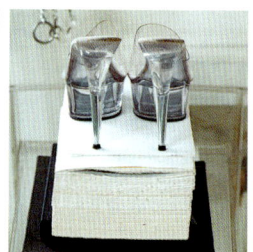

Designer **Pamela Daniels**
Commissioning editor **Annabel Morgan**
Location researcher **Tracy Ogino**
Production **Gemma Moules**
Art director **Anne-Marie Bulat**
Publishing director **Alison Starling**

Stylist **Lorraine Dawkins**

First published in the U.S.
in 2006 by Ryland Peters & Small
519 Broadway, 5th Floor
New York, NY 10012
www.rylandpeters.com

10 9 8 7 6 5 4 3 2 1
Printed in China

Text, design, and photographs
© Ryland Peters & Small 2006

All rights reserved. No part of this publication may be reproduced, stored in a retrieval system, or transmitted in any form or by any means, electronic, mechanical, photocopying, or otherwise, without the prior permission of the publisher.

ISBN-10: 1-84597-262-7
ISBN-13: 978-1-84597-262-2

contents

introduction	6
history of the hcel	8
dressed for success	18
grown-up glamour	28
sense and sensuality	40
special occasions	50
business credits	62
picture credits and acknowledgments	64

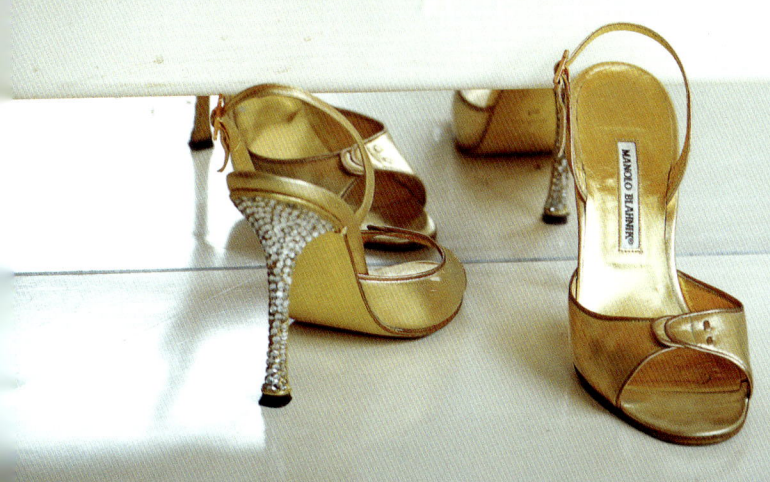

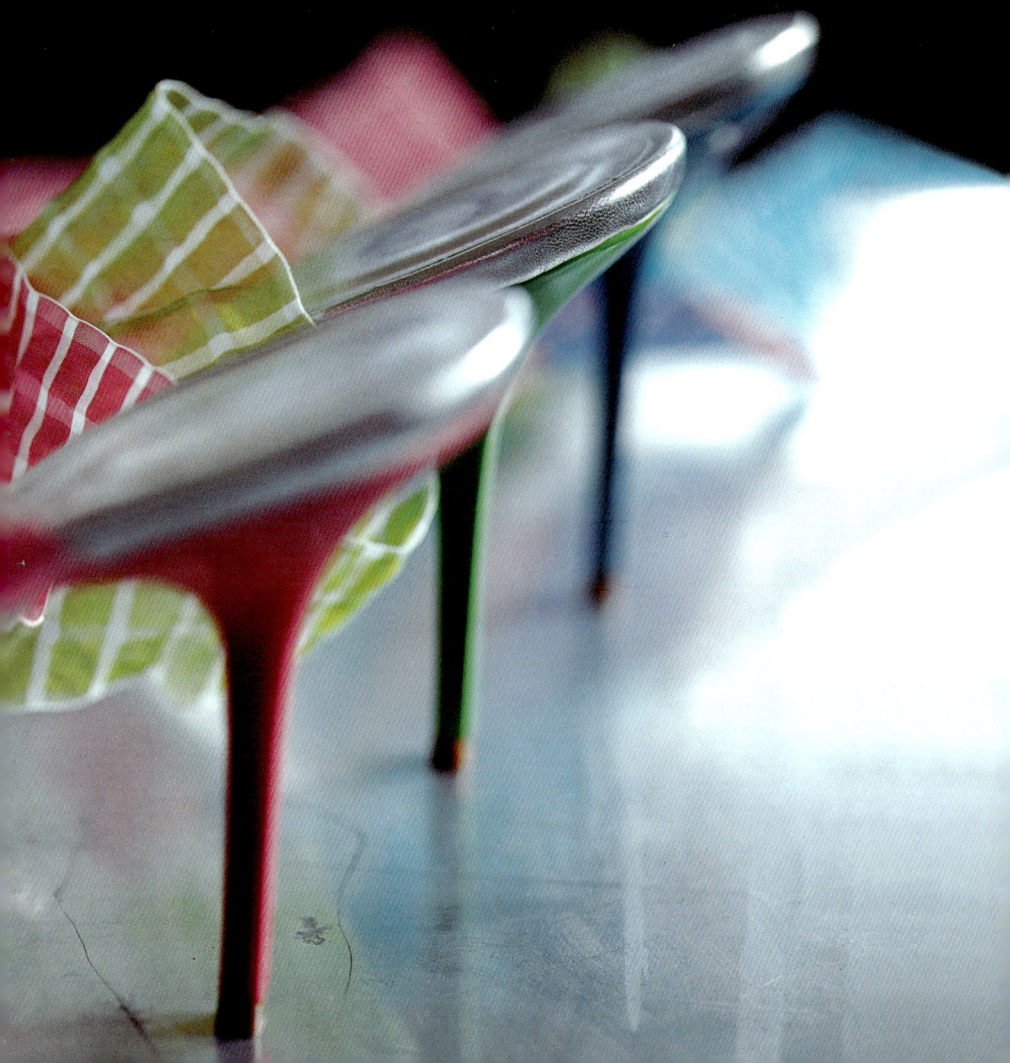

introduction

Shoes tell stories. Shoes trigger memories. Shoes become part of us: they take on the spirit of our lives. In turn, we behave differently to live up to our shoes.

> "...the maiden's left slipper remained sticking. The King's son picked it up, and it was small and dainty, and all golden."
>
> FROM *CINDERELLA* BY JACOB GRIMM (1785–1863) AND WILHELM GRIMM (1786–1859)

Stilettos are sexy. Put on a pair of stilettos, and the transformation is dramatic. They add inches to our height and take inches off our body. They tilt us at a more flattering angle, thrusting the sexiest parts of our bodies up and out.

The love affair with heels starts when we are young. Storybooks tell of the magic powers of shoes. Cinderella's glass slipper and Dorothy's ruby shoes capture our imagination and make our toes curl with pleasure long before we're old enough to experience the heady rush of guilt-edged shoe shopping.

Be warned: when you see the perfect pair of stilettos, you'll be in the red, and head over heels in love. And what's really dangerous is this: it's perfectly okay to be in love with more than one pair of stilettos at the same time.

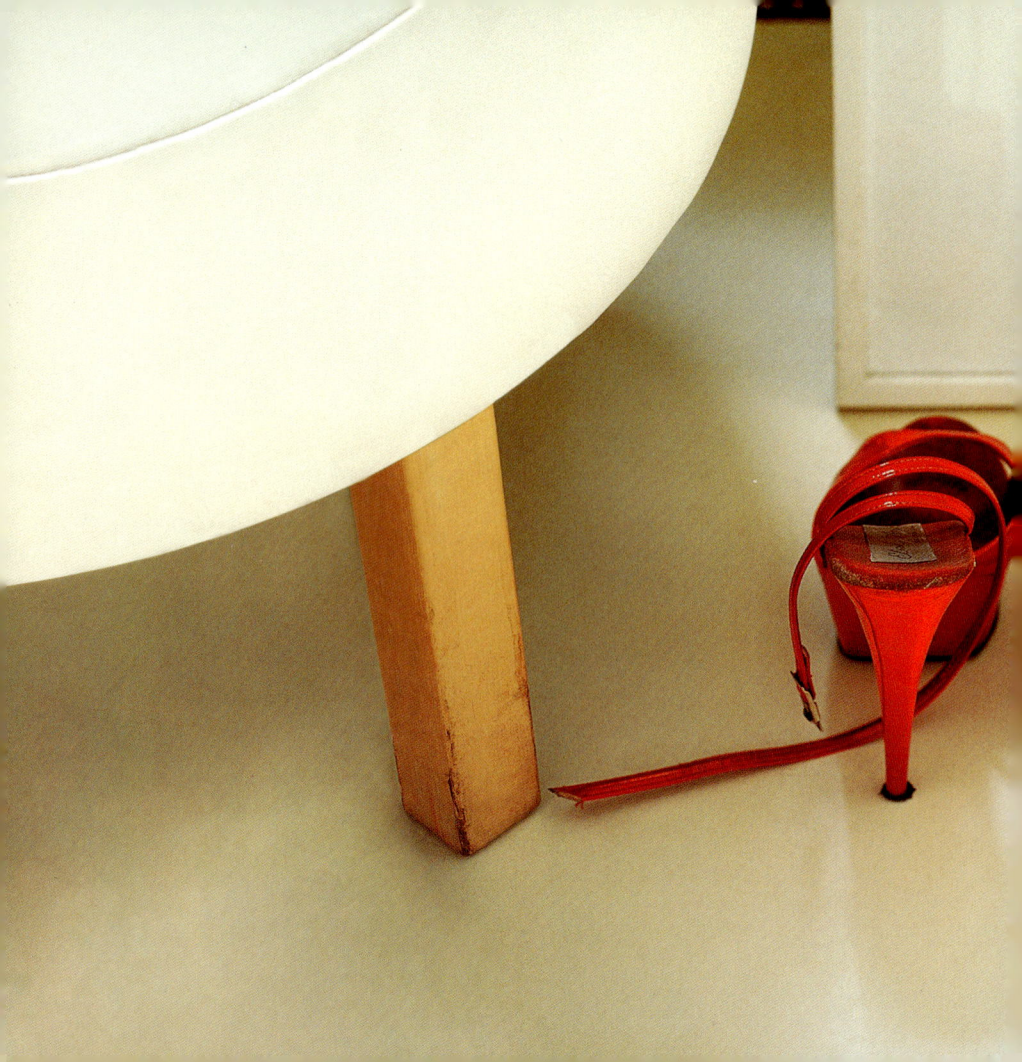

HISTORY OF THE HEEL

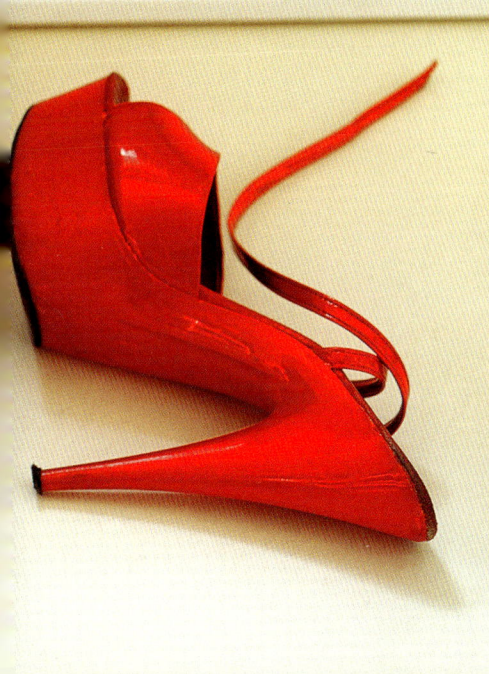

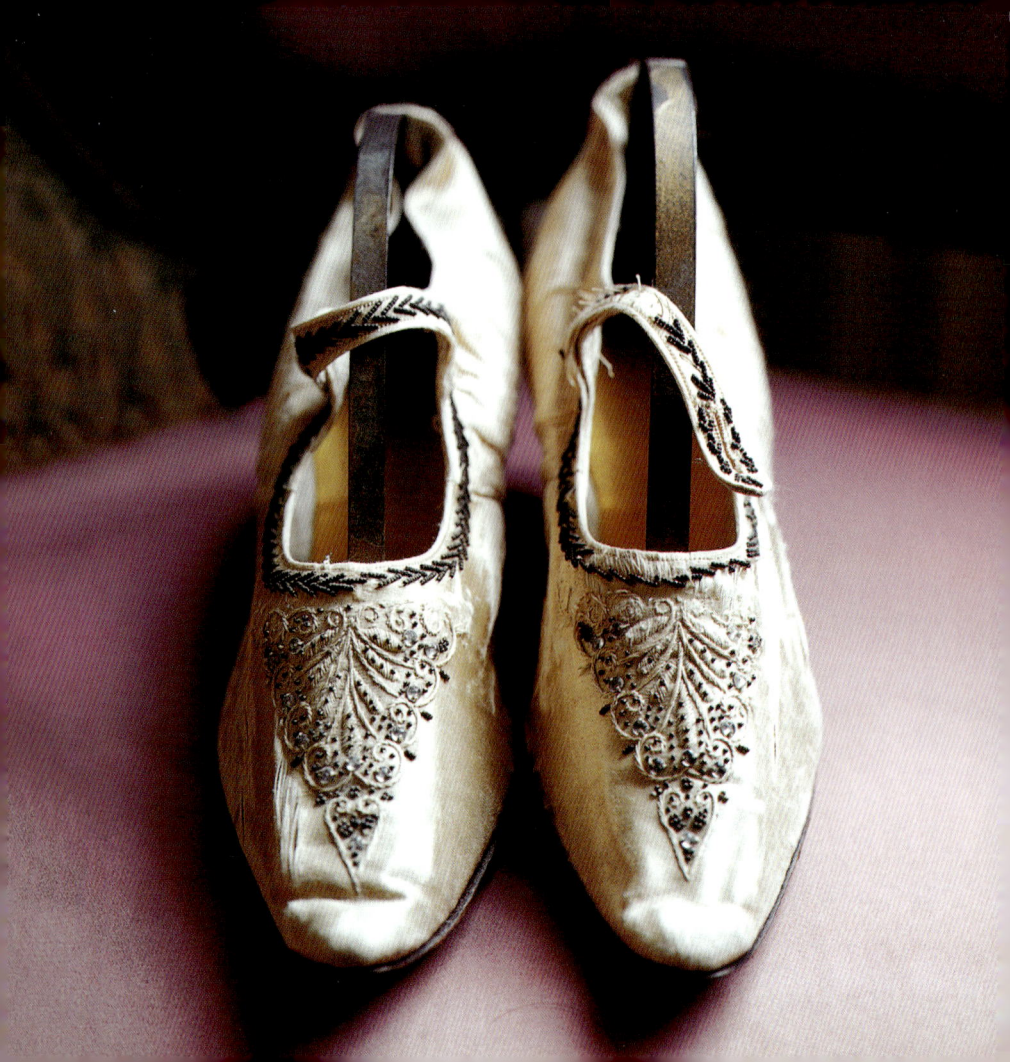

history of the heel

> *"I don't know who invented the high heel, but all women owe him a lot."*
>
> MARILYN MONROE
> (1926–1962)

Leonardo da Vinci is often credited with the invention of the high heel. You might expect such a creative genius to be the brains behind such an elevated invention, but in fact heels had already crept up a notch long, long before Leonardo was at work. In pre-Christian times, Egyptian butchers favored high heels as a way of raising themselves above the carnage, while at the beginning of the 16th century Mongolian horseriders had heels put on their boots in order to get a better grip on their stirrups, making high heels high fashion for men.

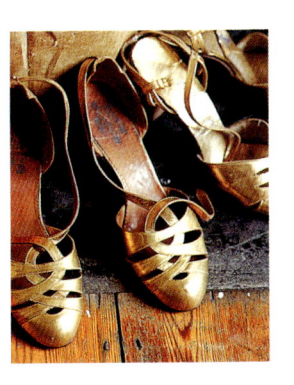

When the 14-year-old Catherine de Medici married the Duke of Orleans in 1533, she opted for modest two-inch heels to walk up the aisle. Next up were chopines, precipitous pedestals in cork or wood, some as tall as 30 inches, and popular with Italian, French, and Spanish women in the mid-1500s. Ladies in Venice needed two maids to help them get in and out of a gondola. At the same time in England, brides who tried this trick were likely to have their marriage annulled if their husbands found out.

> *"It is alleged indeed, that the high heels are most agreeable to our ancient constitution: but however this be, his Majesty hath determined to make use of only low heels in the administration of the government."*
>
> FROM *GULLIVER'S TRAVELS* BY JONATHAN SWIFT (1667–1745)

Two hundred years later or thereabouts, Marie Antoinette ascended to the guillotine wearing fashionable two-inch heels. Before the French Revolution, the "Louis" heel (named after Louis XV) had come into vogue; often as high as five inches tall and highly decorated. After the Revolution, high heels lost their lofty aspirations and fell from favor.

When Queen Victoria came to the throne in 1837, the mood in dress was sober. Women were encouraged to make their feet look small and dainty, and satin flats became popular. By the 1850s, low heels were back in fashion, but only ten years later they had risen to about two and a half inches. The low-heeled mule design later segued into the modern dress pump.

In the late 19th century, it was a case of "Going down: crinolines;" "Going up: back bustles." The season's must-have was a pair of high-heeled boots to show your bustle at its best. The "Grecian bend" was the desired posture: ladies bent forward and stuck out their behinds, while keeping their backs straight.

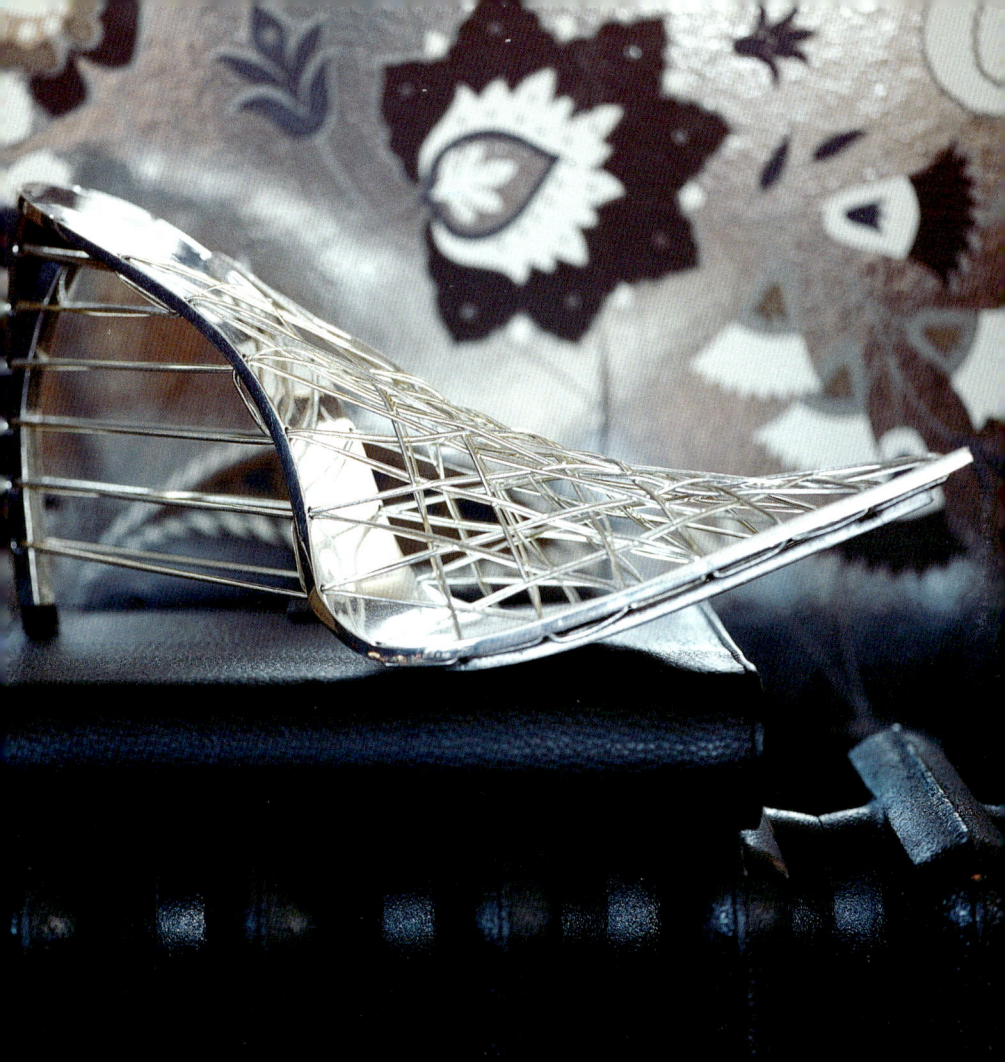

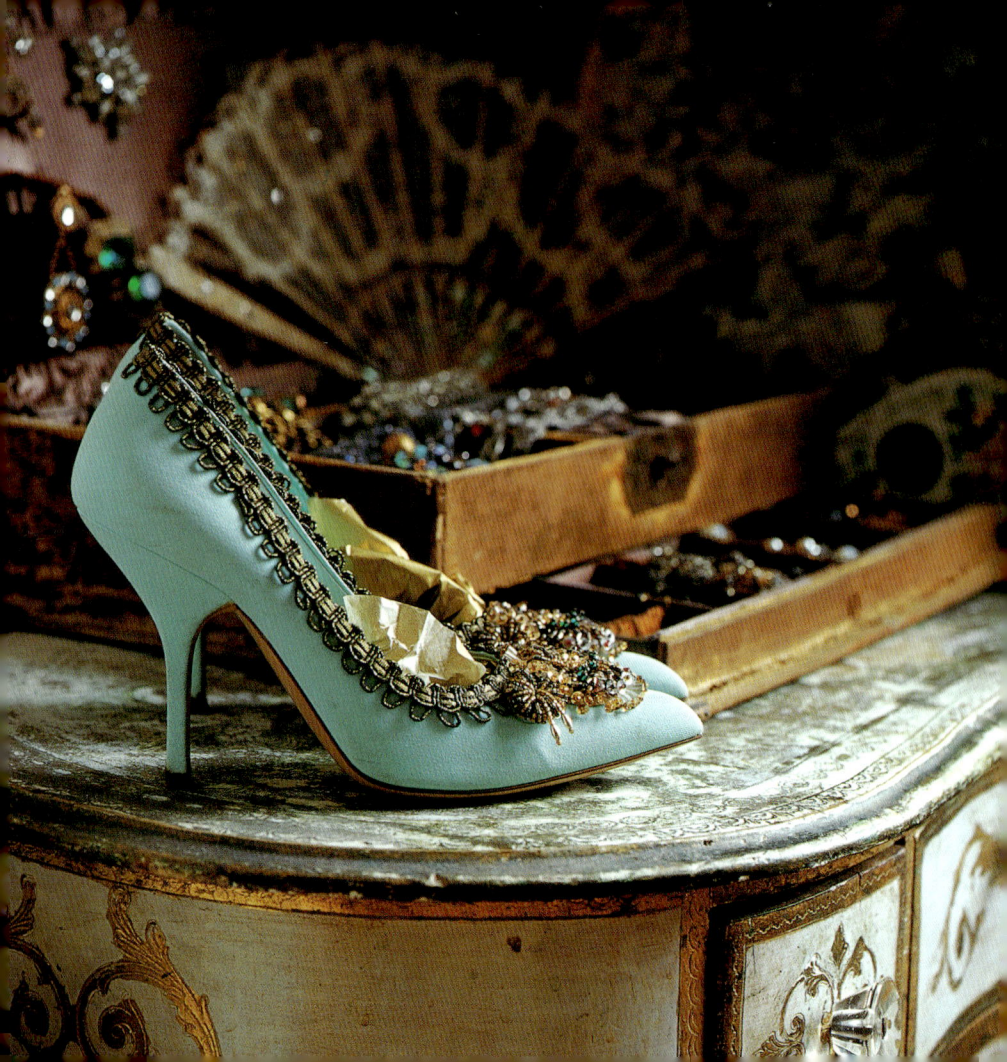

And then, in the early 1950s, the stiletto heel, also known as the needle, rapier, or spike, arrived in France. Or was it Italy? Nobody can quite agree where this new trend began its life. Roger Vivier, a designer who had his toe in the door of Dior at just the right time, is most often credited with designing the first stiletto. Yet many other designers—Salvatore Ferragamo, Charles Jourdan, and Andre Perugia—were also toiling away in their studios, with the tall order of raising women's expectations with a precariously heady construction.

Cobblers around the globe rejoiced in the new trend: the metal stiletto heel tip would need regular replacements. Doctors warned of the damage that heels of such

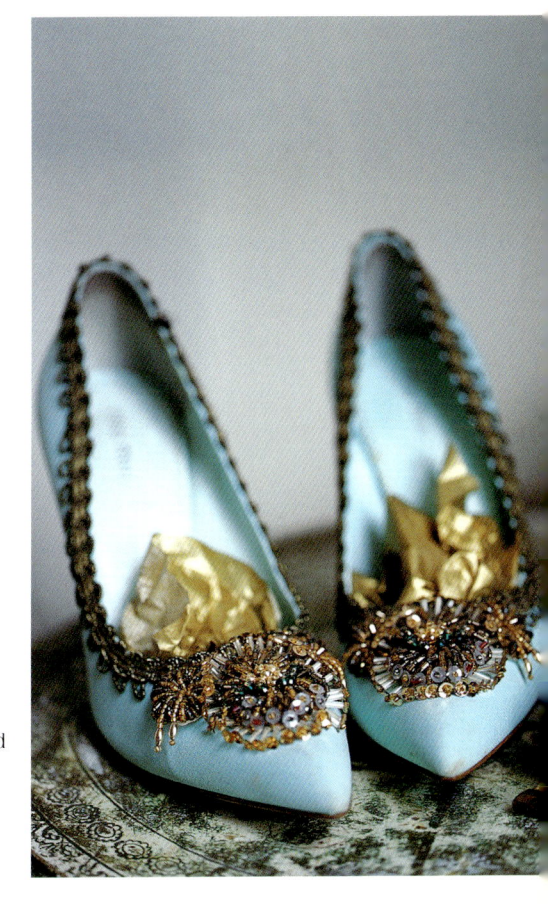

"Light she was and like a fairy, And her shoes were number nine, Herringboxes without topses, Sandals were for Clementine."

FROM *CLEMENTINE* BY PERCY MONTROSS (19TH CENTURY)

a height could do to the posture, while others worried about their polished floors. But women (and men!) were seduced by stilettos and their effect on the female figure: they arch the back, seem to lengthen the calves and spine, and thrust the chest forward.

The stiletto heel started its life in wood, but during the 20th century designers began to experiment with other materials. Borrowing techniques from architecture and aeronautical engineering, prototype stiletto heels were created from materials such as steel alloy and aluminum. In the 1950s, stiletto designers were groundbreaking engineers: Mehmet Kurdash, the founder of the renowned shoe company Gina (named after his favorite actress, Gina Lollobrigida) reinforced a wooden heel with an aluminum spigot, and contemporary stilettos still use this structure. Today, shoes by the revered Manolo Blahnik and his contemporaries are rarely seen as mere footwear—they are more often appreciated as sensual sculptures and coveted works of art. As Roger Vivier said, "To wear dreams on one's feet is to begin to give reality to one's dreams."

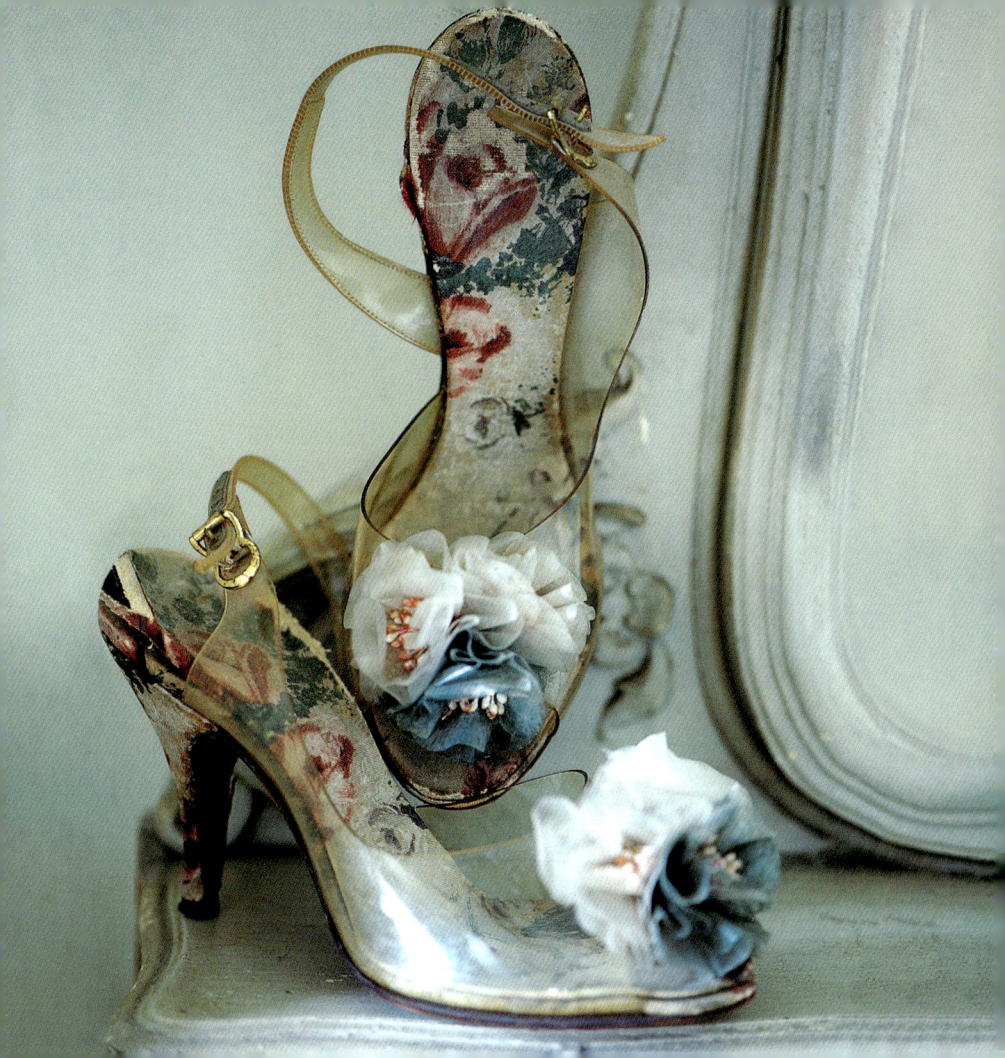

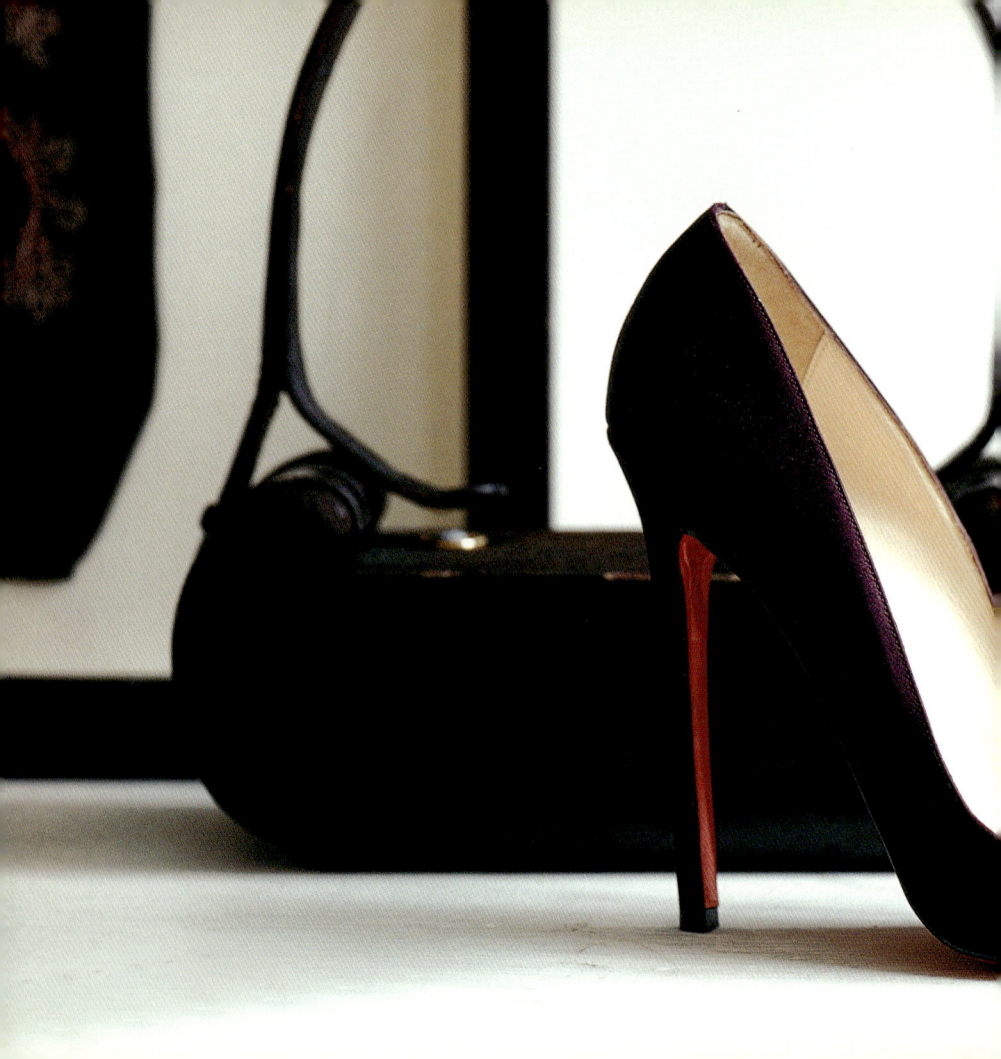

DRESSED FOR SUCCESS

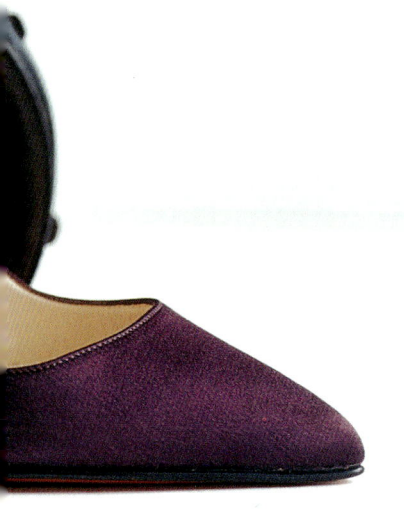

well-heeled

In the interview for the job of your dreams, the decision is made in the first three seconds. Allegedly. This may well be a case of "If the face fits," but, frankly, you can only enhance your chances of success by observing the 18th-century saying, "If the shoe fits, wear it." Stiletto heels will give you a leg up in the world.

Height has always been synonymous with power. Not for nothing did Louis XV wear five-inch heels—some of them decorated with miniature battle scenes—and during his reign high "Louis" heels also became fashionable for women.

When Margaret Thatcher was in power, the climate for women in business was to show they meant business. Suits were sharp, colors were sober, and shirts were tailored. Shoulder pads signaled that the wearer was not to be messed with. As for heels? They were known as killer heels. The spikes might have been to demonstrate that they could smash their way through the glass ceiling or trample over anyone who happened to be in their path. Skirts got shorter

"Be sure you put your feet in the right place, then stand firm."

ABRAHAM LINCOLN
(1809–1865)

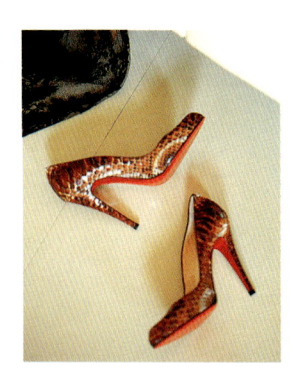

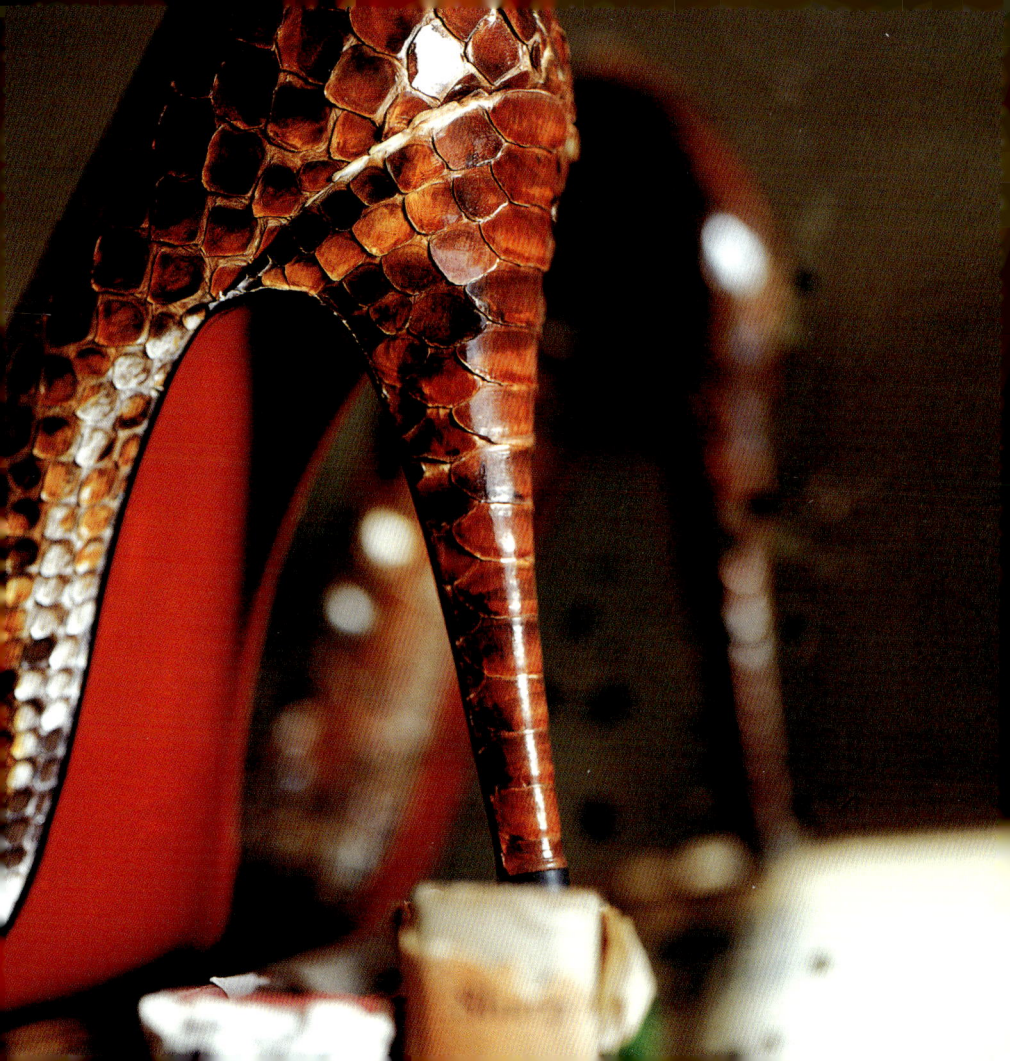

manolo blahnik drawings

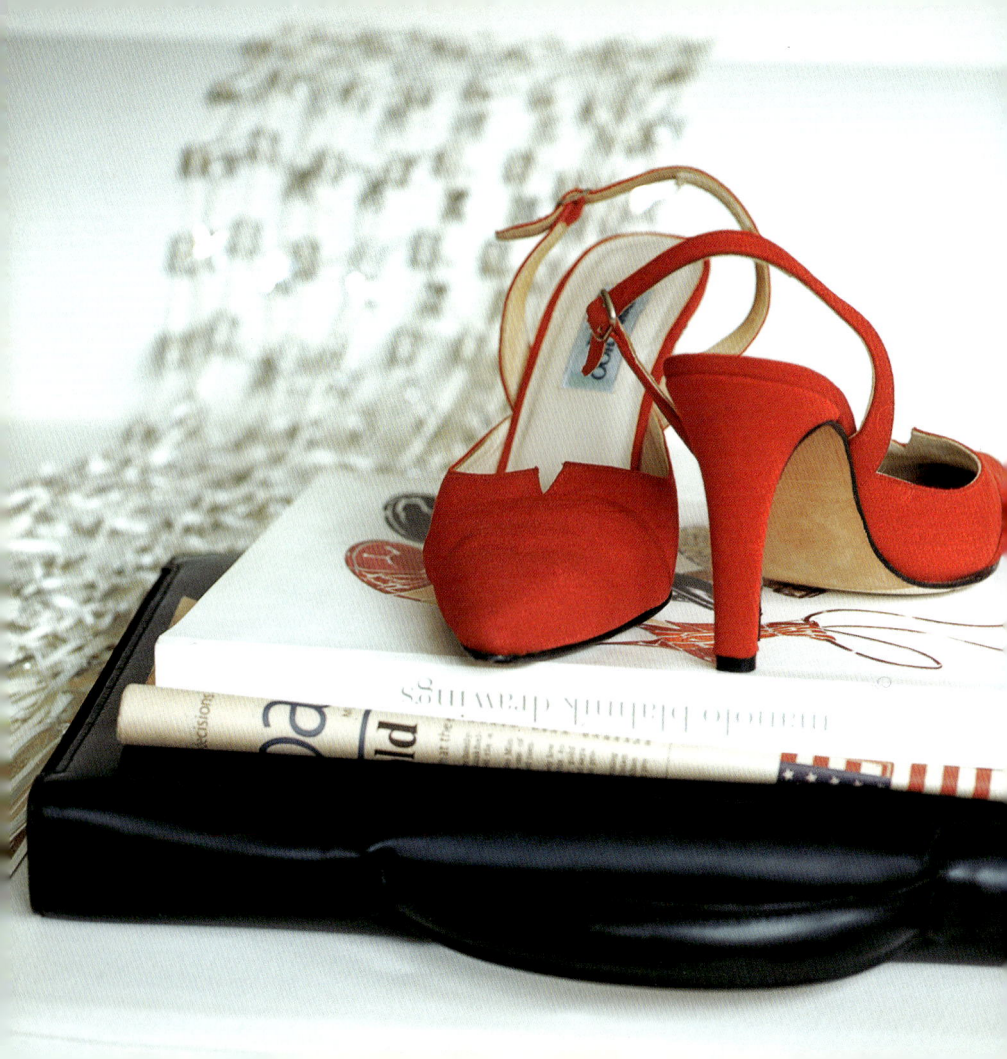

and heels got spikier, yet some women still managed to emit an aura of vulnerability and femininity. It was a confused and competitive world. Needless to say, this style of dress didn't really help if you were late for work. Melanie Griffith, keen to cast off her comfy sneakers and shoehorn her feet into killer heels for the office in the film *Working Girl*, created a trend for women to walk to work in their sneakers—something that continues to this day.

Thankfully, the knockout shoulder pads sported by the heroines in *Dallas* and *Dynasty* are long gone, but the reality is that, while needle heels were a symbol of authority during the decade of power dressing, spikes still spell success.

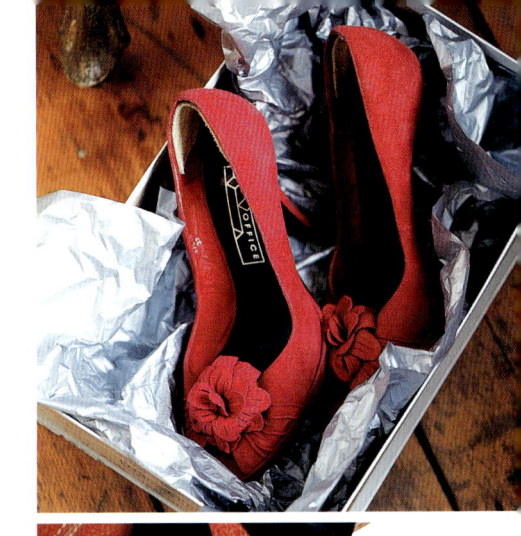

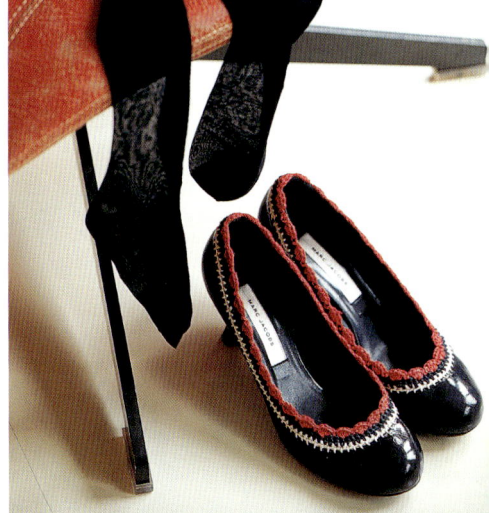

best foot forward

> *"Ambition has one heel nailed in well, though she stretches her fingers to touch the heavens."*
>
> LAO-TZU
> (6TH CENTURY B.C.)

You're having a bad hair day. You feel like putting on a slouchy sweater, staying in, shuffling around, perhaps watching a soap. You might be slightly grumpy and feeling sorry for yourself. "Poor me," says your inner victim. Now kick off your flip-flops, slippers, or whatever you've been slumping around in. Stand in front of a full-length mirror, put on your Manolos (or your favorite pair of heels) and take a look. You will have metamorphosed into a winner.

It's a bit like doing a room makeover. You buy a new lampshade, then all of a sudden the rest of the room looks shabby and you have to completely redecorate. So it is with heels. Step into your spikes, and you'll feel compelled to throw off your sweatpants and sink into a bathful of fragrant bubbles. Then you'll be inspired to do a full pedicure. And look at your hair! That needs washing, too.

When you're up there, teetering high above the detritus of your bedroom floor, it's impossible to feel down. Put your best foot forward and you'll change your whole demeanor

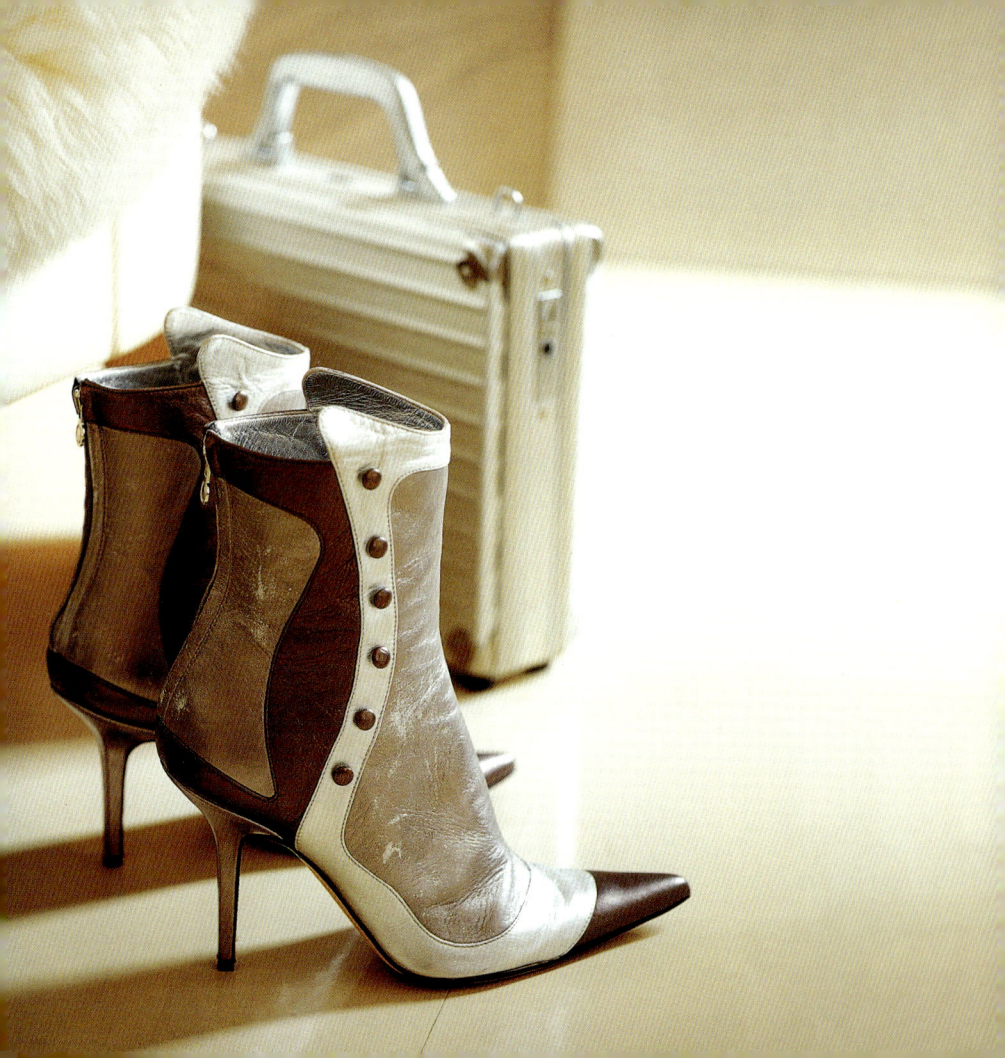

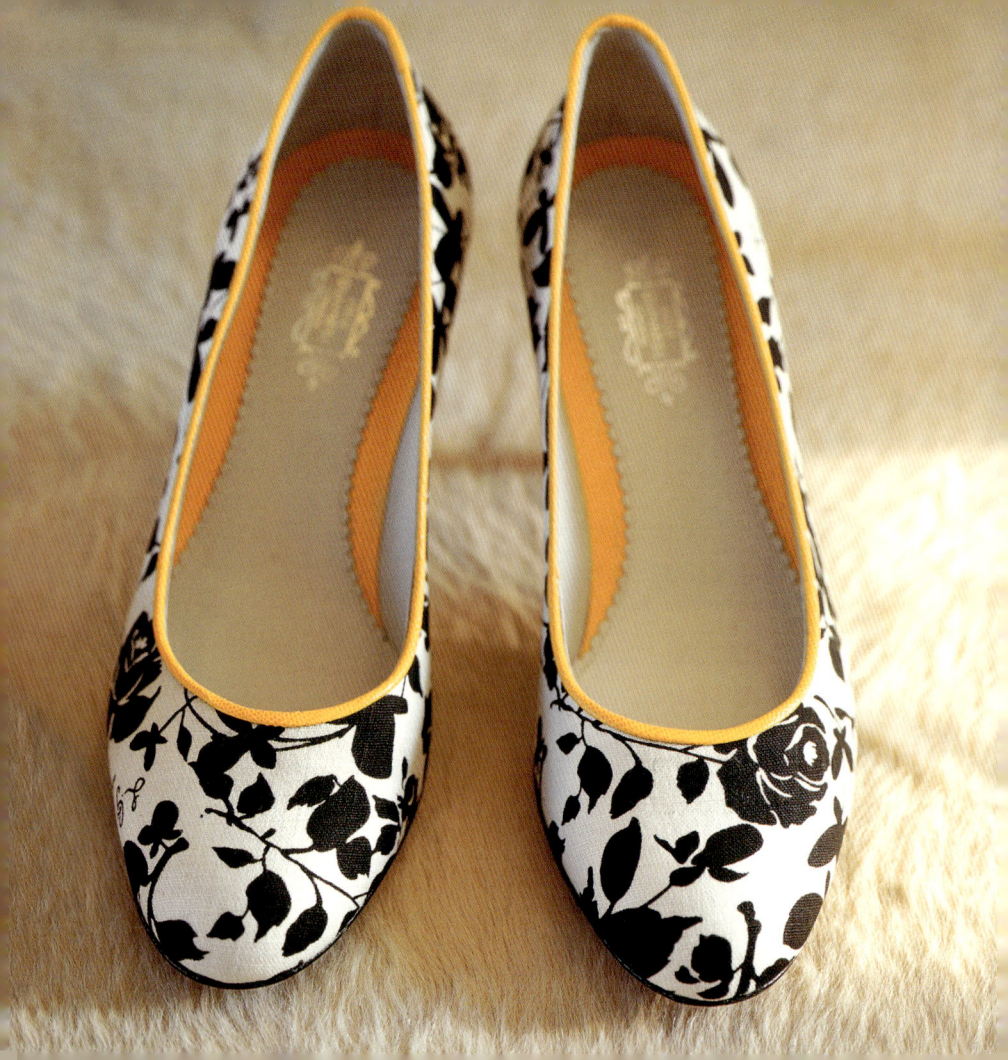

to match your shoes. Before you know it, your hair will be bouncy and you'll walk tall and feel fantastic. It's official—stilettos lift the spirits. You'll breeze into that interview and blow them away. And when you do get your dream job, just think of all the shoes you'll be able to afford … without feeling guilty.

One more thing. High heels focus the mind. You can't afford to look backwards when you're wearing stilettos. You need every ounce of concentration just to proceed with a smile on your face and avoid cobblestones, drains, or uneven sidewalk situations. You will find yourself entering a meditative state, becoming grounded and serene. So really you should think of putting on heels as dressing for happiness.

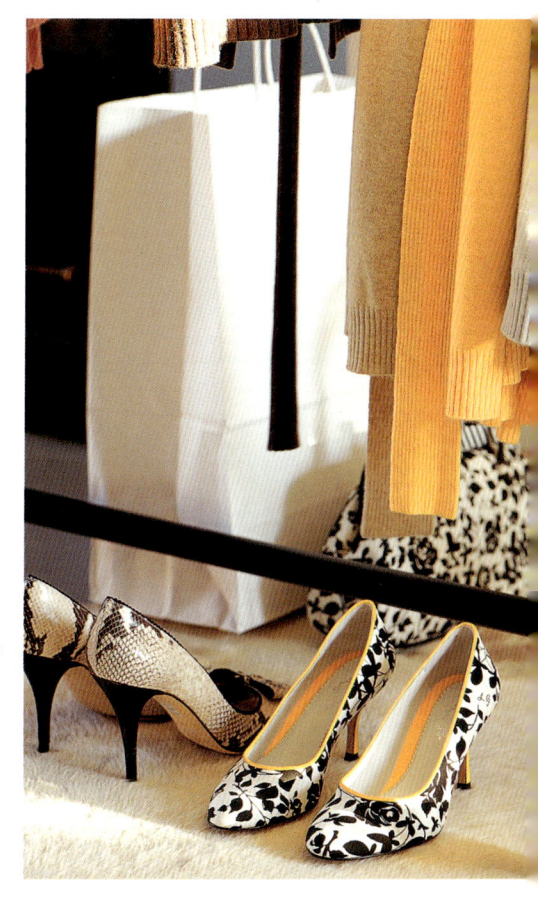

DRESSED FOR SUCCESS 27

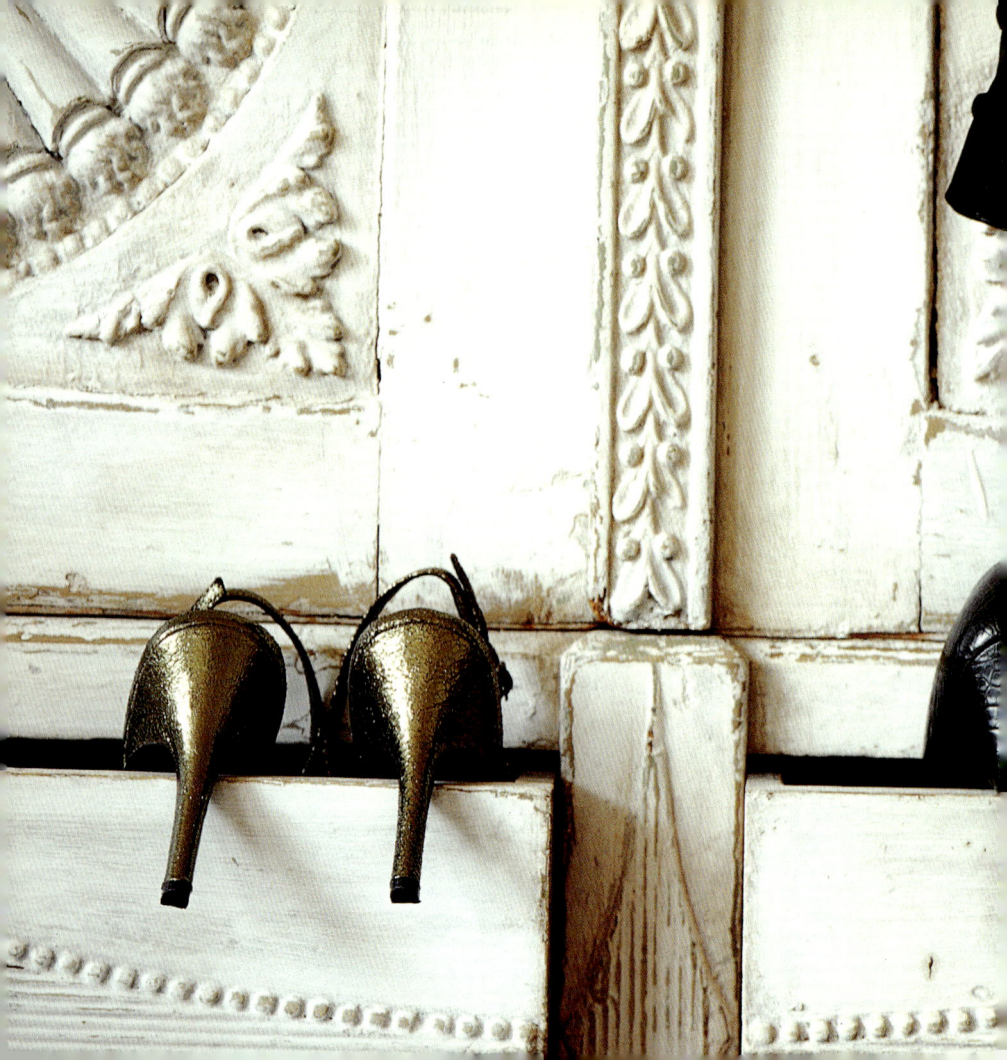

GROWN-UP GLAMOUR

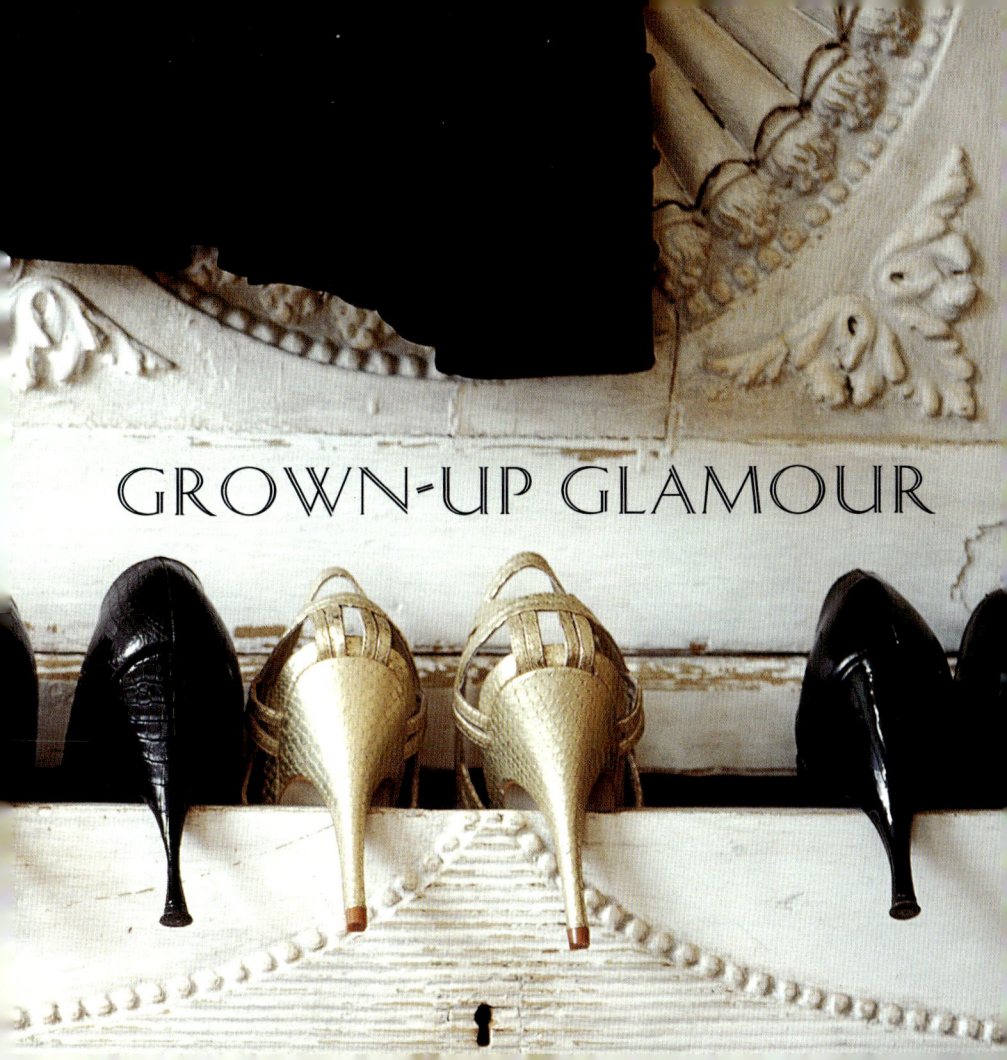

spiked with danger

> *"The imagination is the spur of delight... all depends upon it, it is the mainspring of everything; now, is it not by means of the imagination one knows joy? Is it not of the imagination that the sharpest pleasures arise?"*
>
> MARQUIS DE SADE
> (1740–1814)

Think about it. Would the tension and glamour of *Vertigo* have been anywhere near as menacing had Kim Novak been roaming around San Francisco in a pair of penny loafers? And what about *The Seven Year Itch*? If Marilyn Monroe's skirt had floated up to reveal a stout pair of walking shoes, would the image still be imprinted on our memory?

Hollywood starlets and sex goddesses of the 1950s had a streak of danger; their stockings and stilettos gave them an edge. These women meant business: they exuded confidence in both their sexuality and their femininity. The likes of Ava Gardner, Lauren Bacall, and Grace Kelly knew just how to wear heels to lift their game, adding glamour and drama to their performances both on and off the silver screen.

For instant womanly glamour, all you need to do is slip on a pair of spike-heeled stilettos, and you'll instantly find yourself in tune with your inner sex goddess.

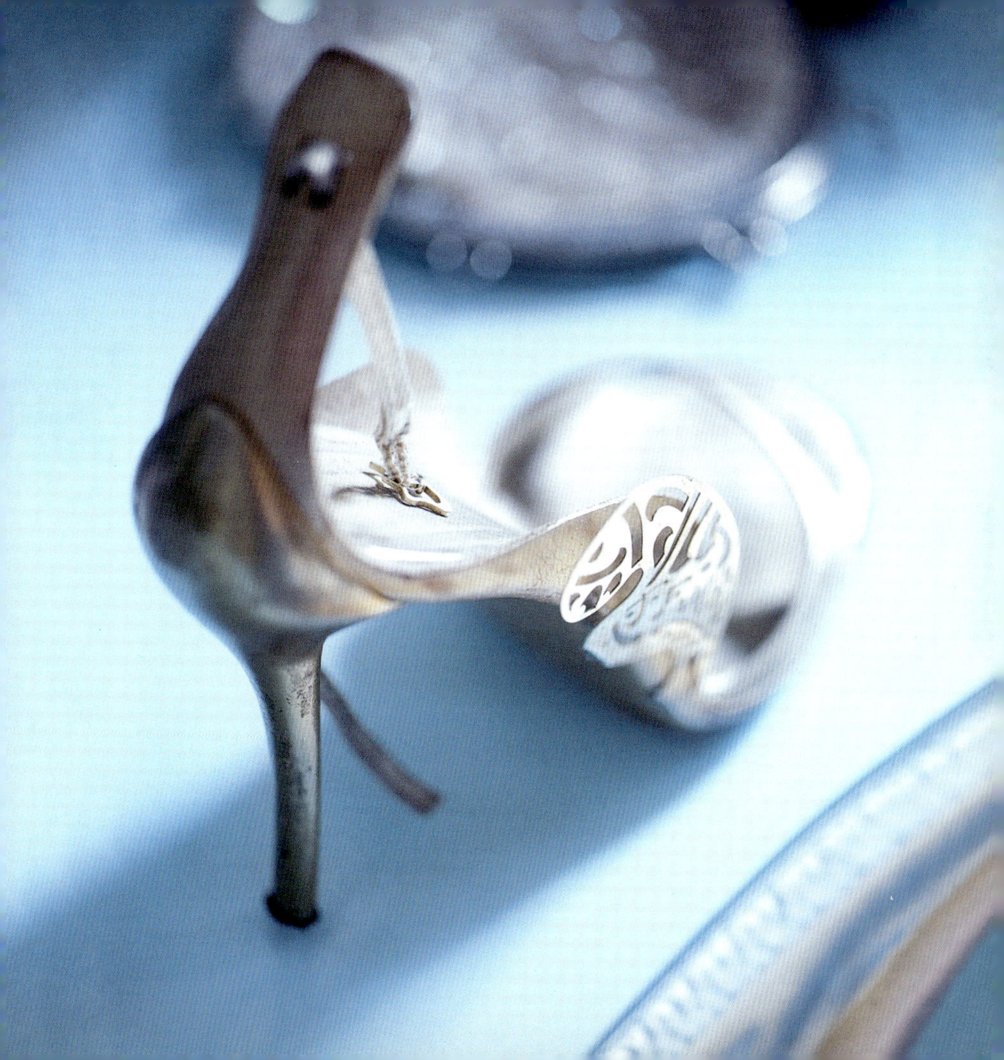

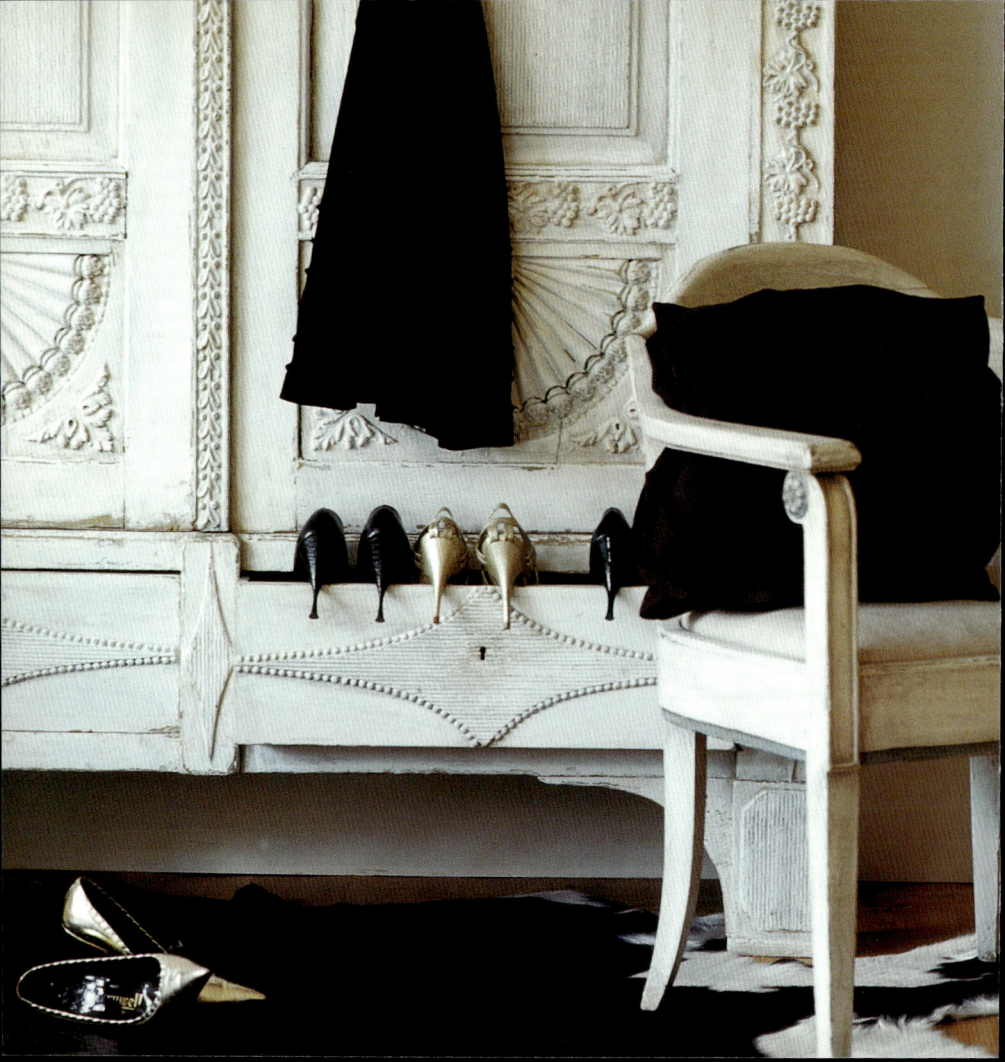

champagne stilettos

During the first golden age of stilettos, in the 1950s, some spike heels were upgraded to the point where they had their own film roles. One memorable stiletto stepped out in Fellini's *La Dolce Vita*, when Anita Ekberg used it to drink champagne from while romping in the Trevi fountain in Rome. And in *High Society*, another stiletto starred alongside Frank Sinatra, who also used it to sip champagne.

Stars of the silver screen formed lasting relationships with the shoe designers of the time. "Ferragamos" in the 1950s were every bit as out there as "Manolos" are today. Just as Sarah Jessica Parker will always be associated with Manolo Blahnik, Marilyn Monroe was known to be a devoted fan of Salvatore Ferragamo.

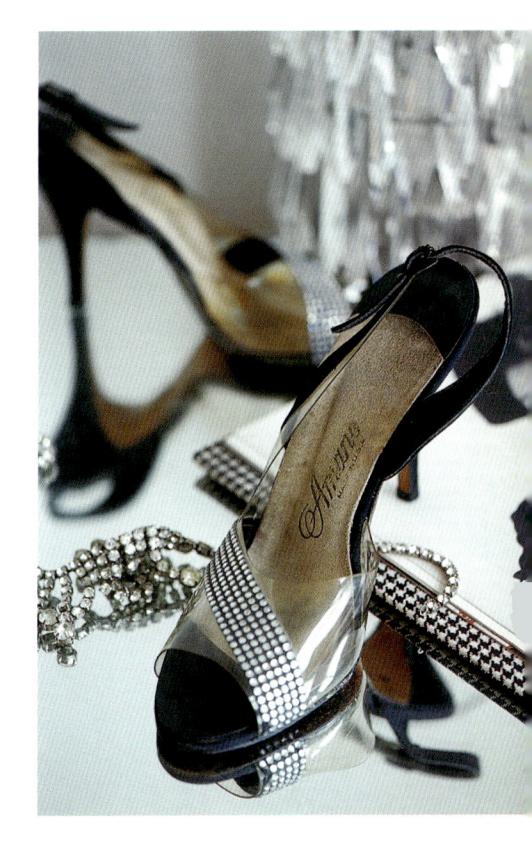

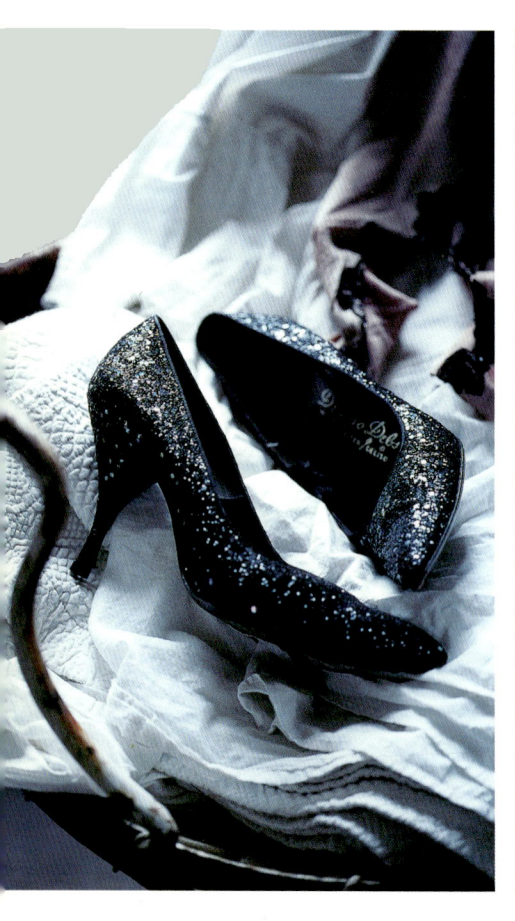

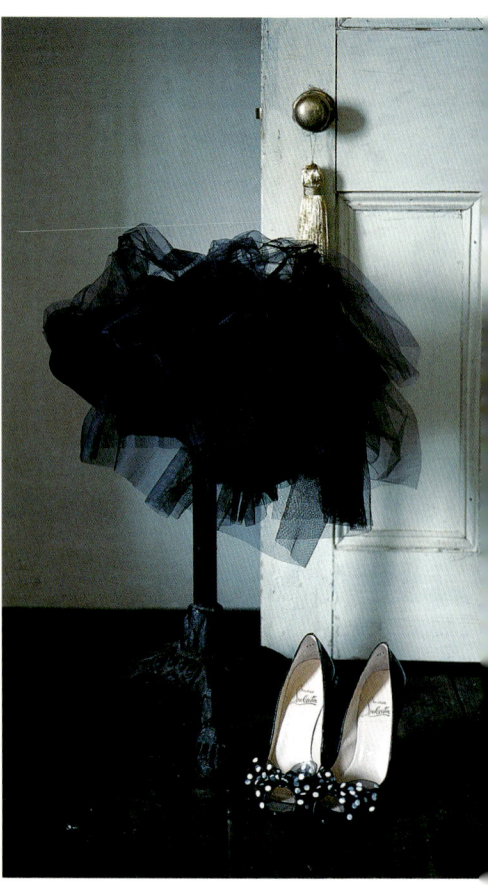

34 GROWN-UP GLAMOUR

In *The Seven Year Itch*, when Marilyn stands above the subway grating, her skirt floats up to reveal a pair of peep-toed, spike-heeled Ferragamo slingbacks. Meanwhile Ava Gardner, star of the 1954 film *The Barefoot Contessa*, adored Roger Vivier's creations for Dior.

Nowadays, stilettos can be foot jewelry. Singer Alison Krauss attended the Oscars one year wearing stiletto sandals encrusted with 500 diamonds set in platinum. The sandals were valued at $2 million. Heels are not only good for tiptoeing through the pile of the red carpet on glittering award nights—diamond and platinum stilettos can also adorn the stars' earlobes. The New York jeweler Harry Winston is famous for his stiletto earrings, which over the years have been worn by Julia Roberts, Holly Hunter, and Charlize Theron.

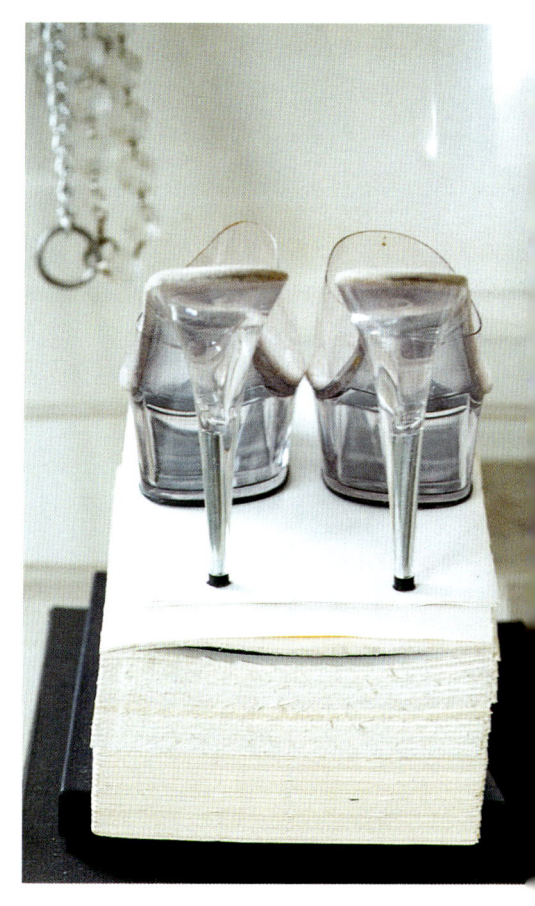

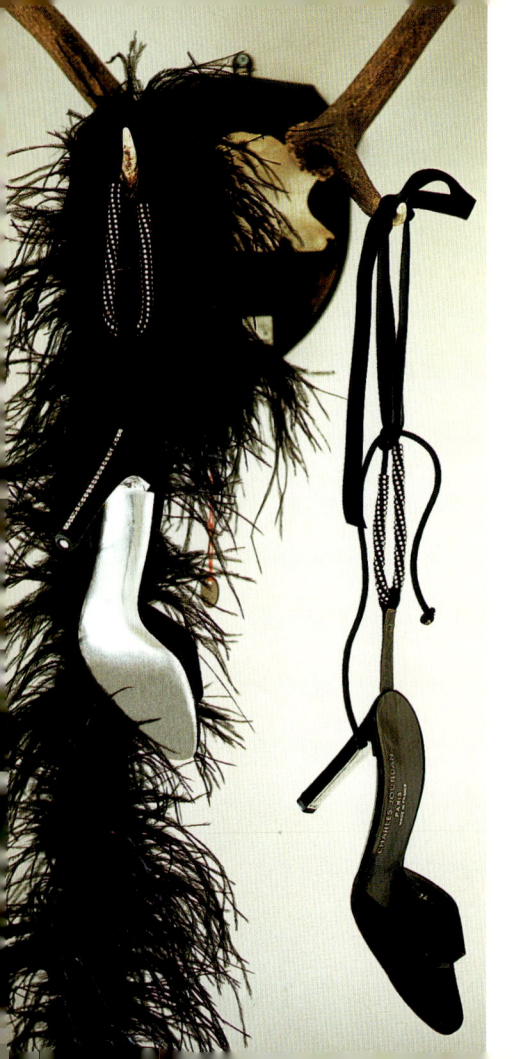

espresso sharp

Named after the Italian stiletto dagger or switchblade, the stiletto heel is tapered and threatening. It gave a dose of daring to both stars and films in Hollywood, but also in Italy, where glamour and style became synonymous with evocative symbols including the Vespa, the Gaggia coffee machine, and needle heels, not to forget the stars themselves, namely Sophia Loren and Gina Lollobrigida.

If you're a Vespa virgin, then now is the time to plan your very own Roman holiday. This doesn't necessarily mean booking a cheap flight for a mini-break (although that is, of course, an option). You can try this out at home. It's really easy. A Vespa is the perfect vehicle, but if you haven't got access to one you'll just have to improvise. Start the day

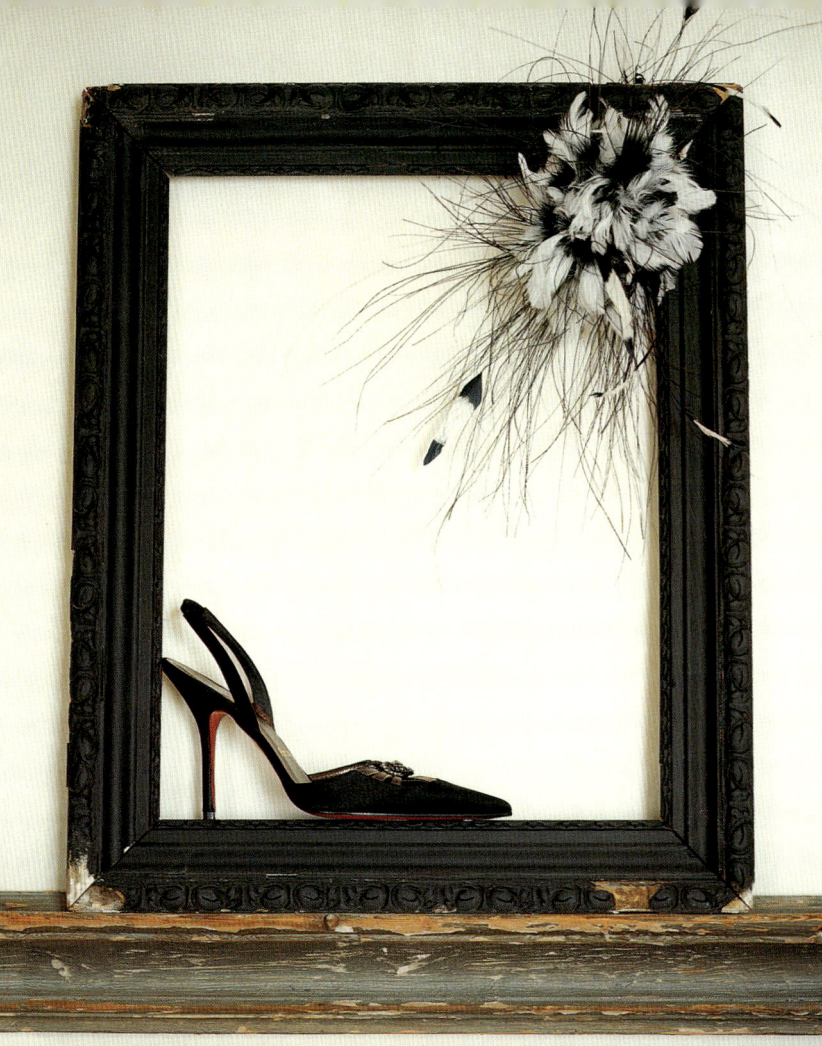

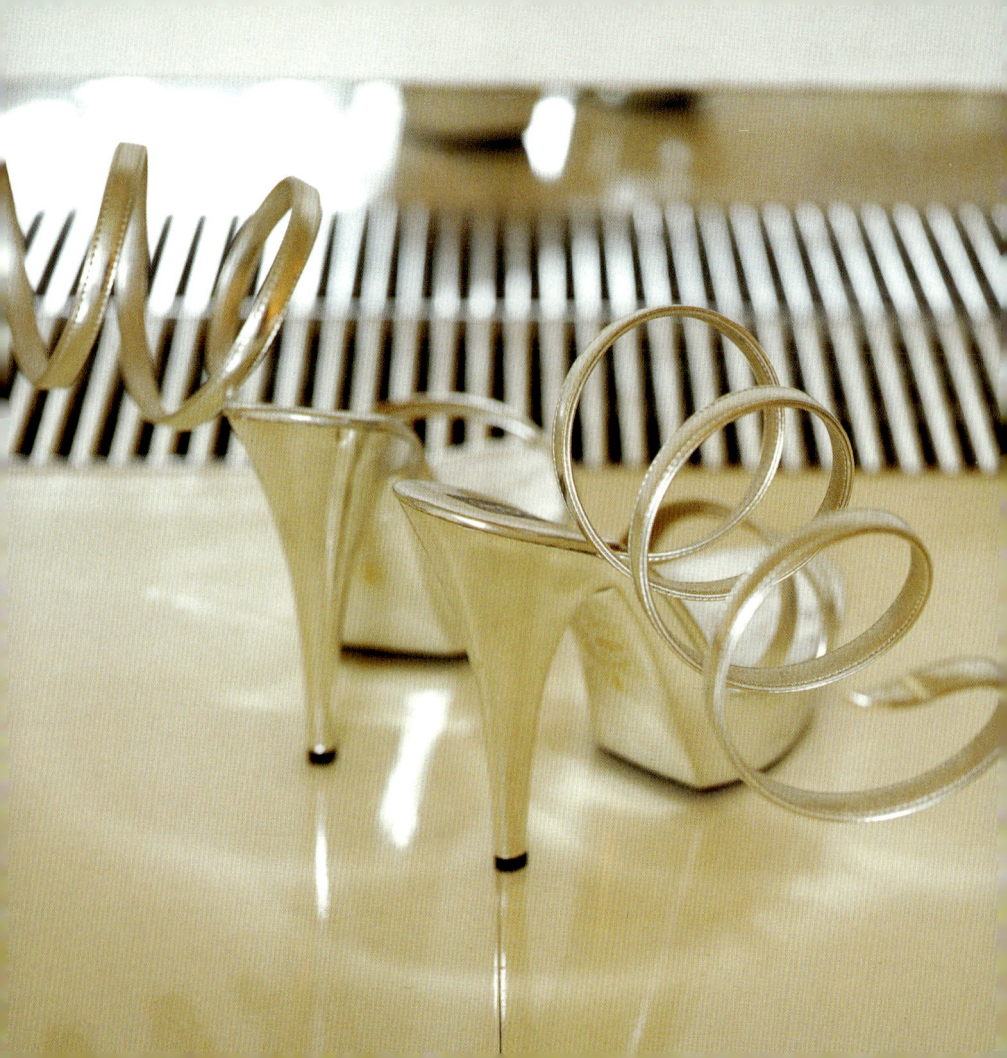

> *"What spirit is so empty and blind, that it cannot recognize the fact that the foot is more noble than the shoe, and skin more beautiful than the garment with which it is clothed?"*
>
> MICHELANGELO BUONARROTI (1475–1564)

with coffee at home—but only if you've got a proper espresso machine. Put on a Verdi CD. Make coffee with lots of hissing noises. Dress as if you'll be stepping out onto cobblestone squares in Rome (although these happen to be a total nightmare with spikes) or as if you'll be riding pillion, buzzing along the Amalfi coast. Wear a sweater—the tighter, the better—or a cinched-in dress with a sticky-out skirt teamed with short white gloves and stilettos.

Sashay with a smile to your local Italian deli. Do some serious hanging out. Cross your legs gracefully and allow one shoe to dangle delicately from your foot. It's not to be recommended, I know, but if you smoke it helps. You can always pop a cigarette in your mouth and pretend you're just about to light it. Hide behind huge sunglasses, and lower them from time to time to smile at any particularly attractive strangers. Download some "Teach Yourself Italian" onto your iPod. Don't drink cappuccino after 10 a.m. if you want to be truly authentic, but it really doesn't matter what you do, as long as you're having lots of fun!

GROWN-UP GLAMOUR

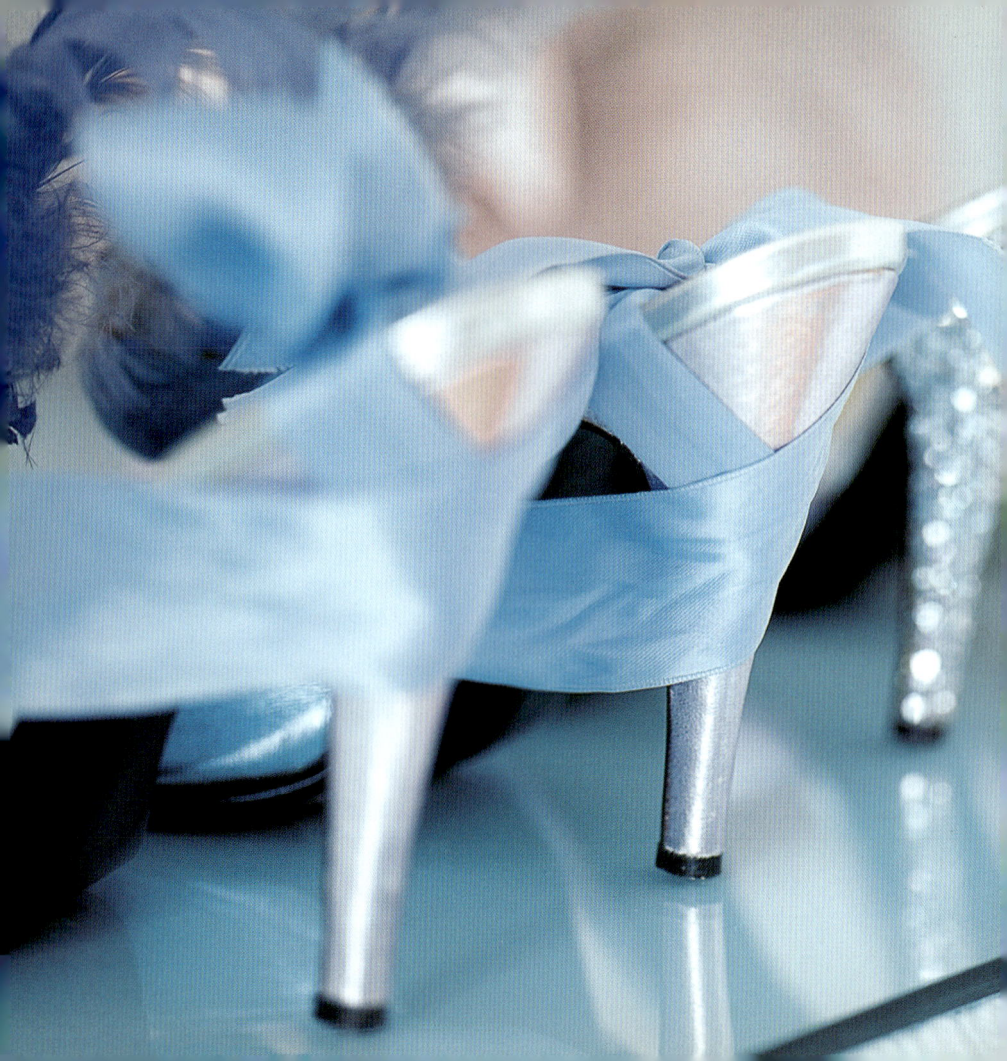

SENSE AND SENSUALITY

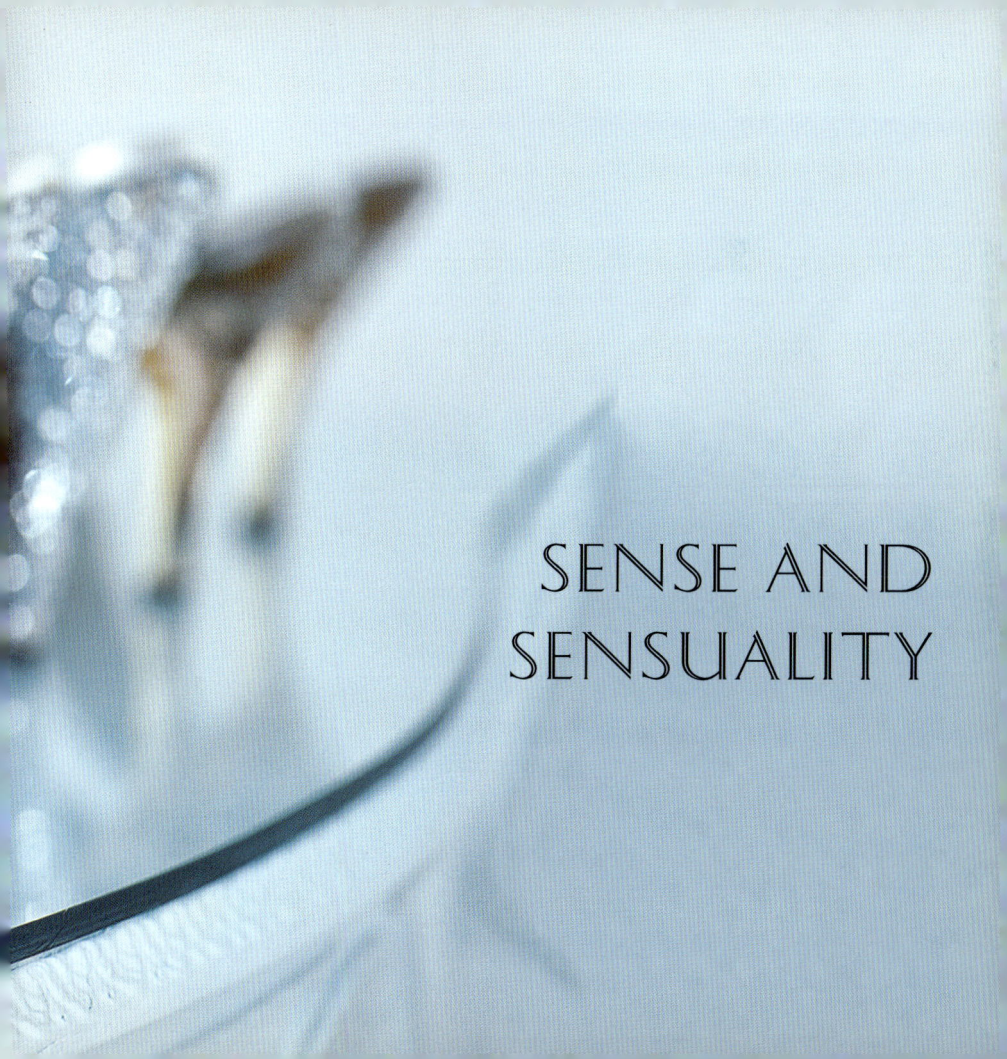

sex and spikes

Stilettos have been associated with sex since the Hollywood cameras were first turned on them. That classic, seductive, and suggestive shot that starts from the heel, moves to the ankle then slides slowly up the leg of Marilyn Monroe, Jayne Mansfield, or Ava Gardner is something you expect to happen before it actually does.

"Opportunity may knock only once, but temptation leans on the doorbell."

ANONYMOUS

A couple of decades later, sex met stilettos head on when the fetish movement enjoyed a revival. Photographers such as Guy Bourdin and Helmut Newton celebrated the sado-masochistic power of spikes. Punks, cross-dressers, and aficionados of disco glam took to their high heels and partied. Debbie Harry was one third of the trashy girl band The Stilettos, who were very much part of the New York punk scene—a mood that she brought with her to Blondie.

Yet by the time Carrie Bradshaw and her friends started wearing them, stilettos were a sign that girls just wanted to have fun. And fun they had. So when you want to get in touch with your sensual side, slip into your spikiest heels.

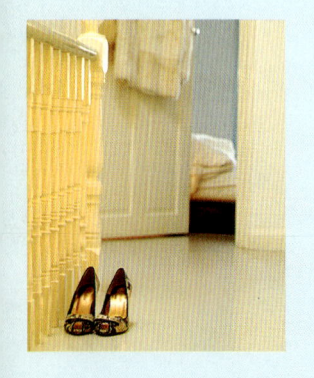

SENSE AND SENSUALITY

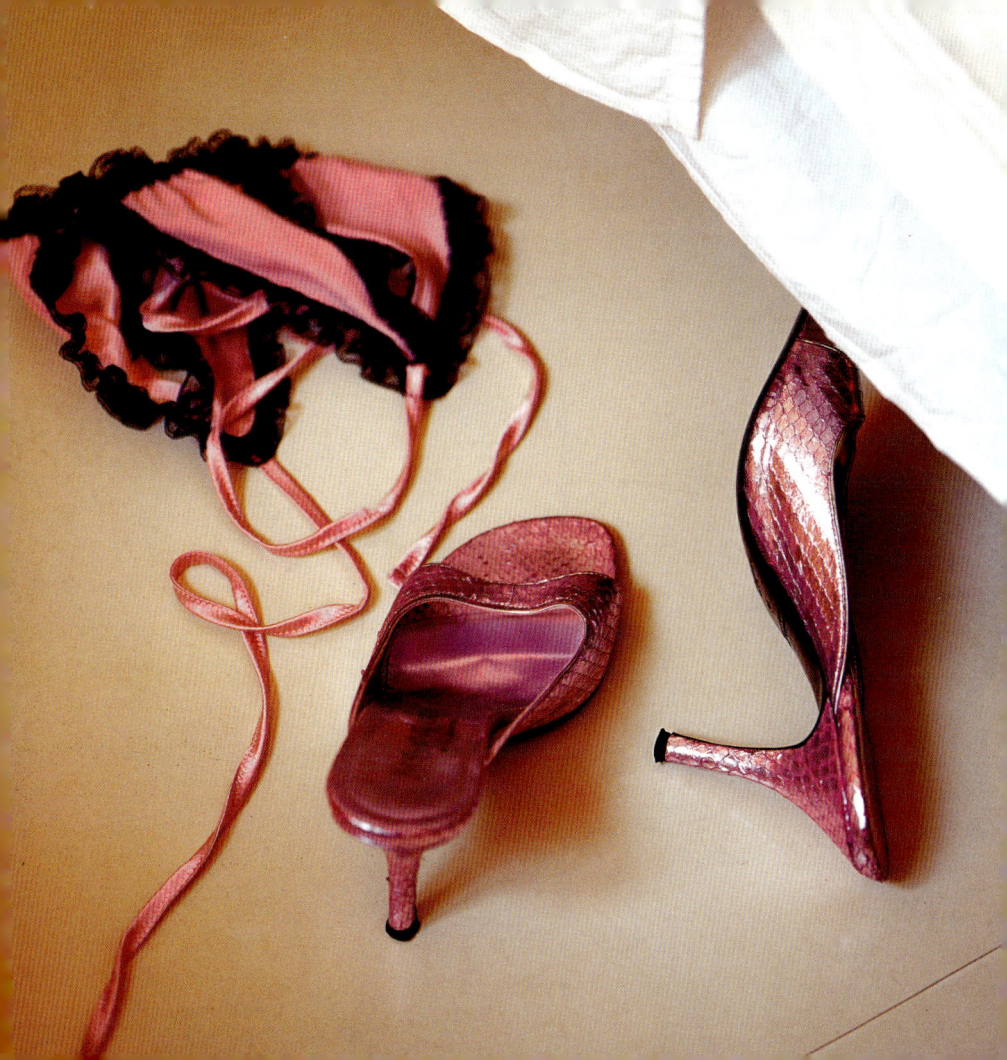

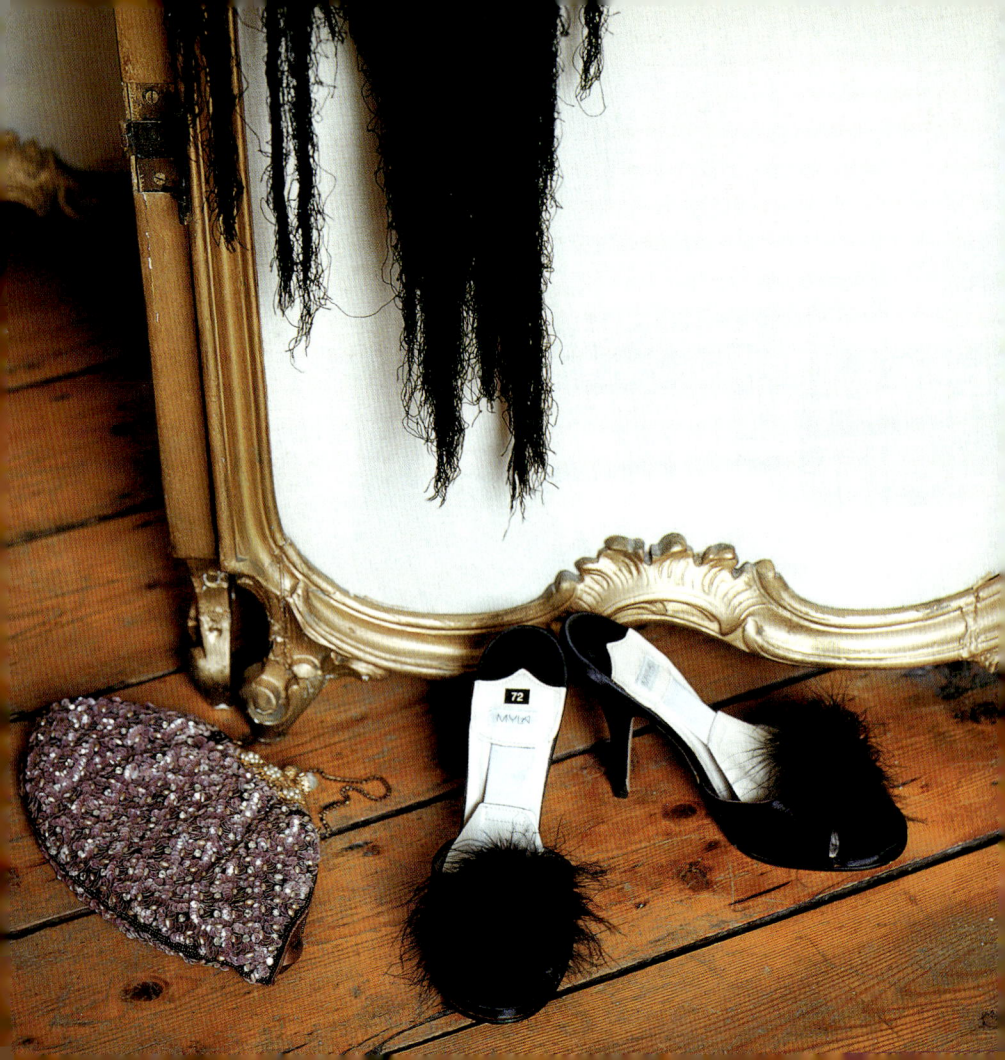

boudoir chic

Just as many of us are modeling our bathrooms on those in hip hotels—with dinner-plate-sized shower heads, perfumed candles, and an abundance of waffle towels and silky body lotions—now is the time to turn our eyes to the bedroom. Forget about sleeping and think about living, in contemporary boudoir chic. Needless to say, stilettos are the perfect footwear for slinky (or even kinky) bedroom behavior, because you're not going to be traveling far.

It's essential to celebrate the fact that "I'm staying in" is clearly not the dreary option. Instead, it's about giving yourself the time and space to be exactly who you want to be—whether you're alone or with your partner.

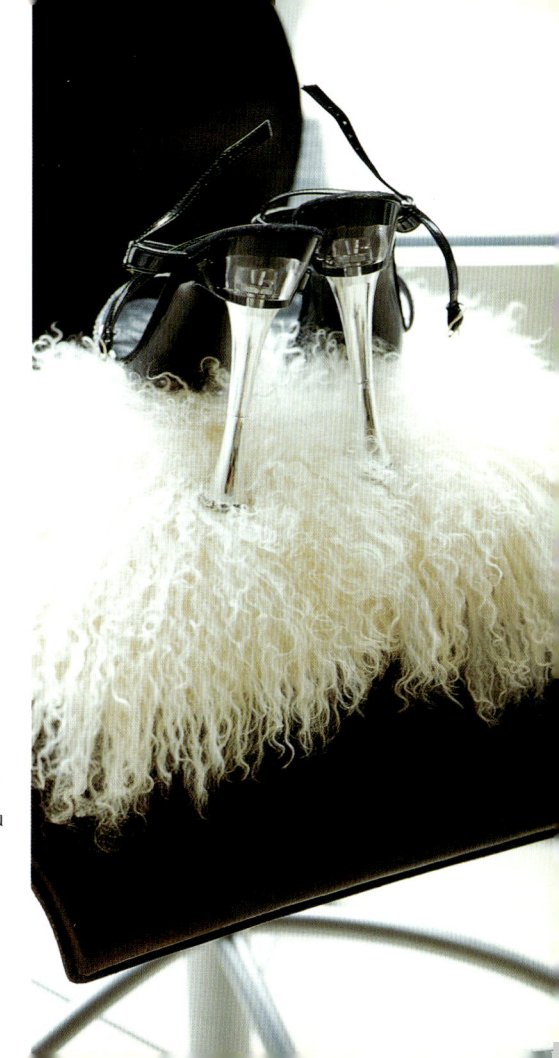

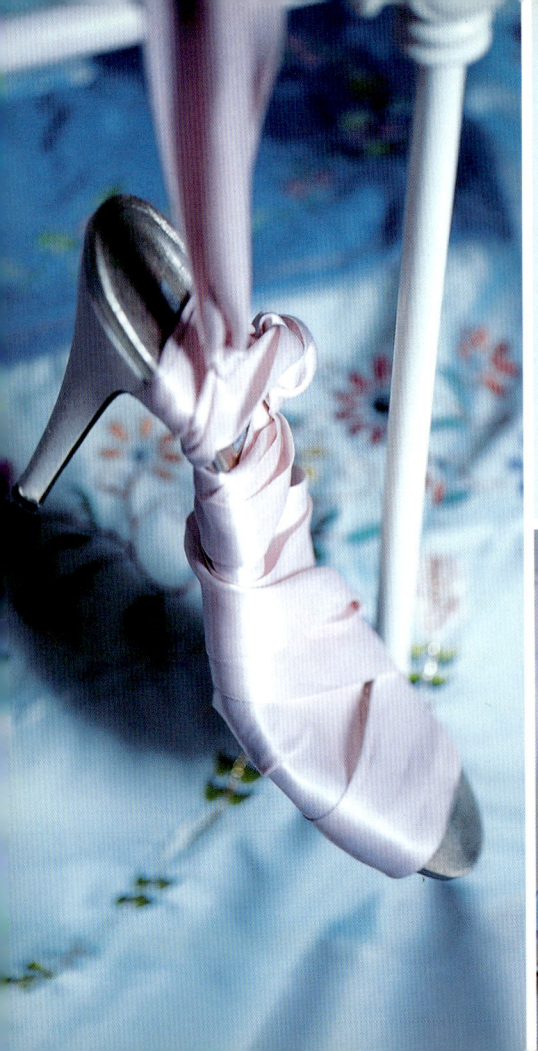

> "There is no unhappier creature on earth than a fetishist who yearns to embrace a woman's shoe and has to embrace the whole woman."

KARL KRAUS (1874–1936)

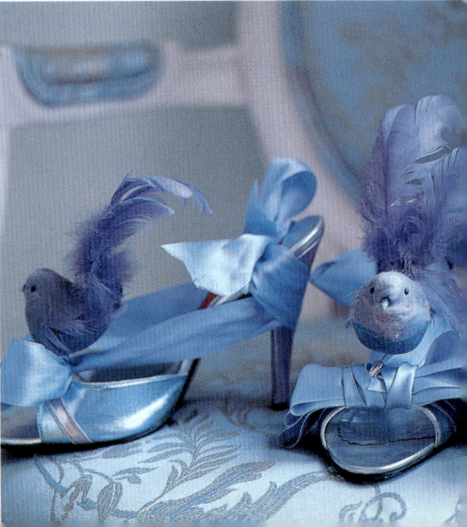

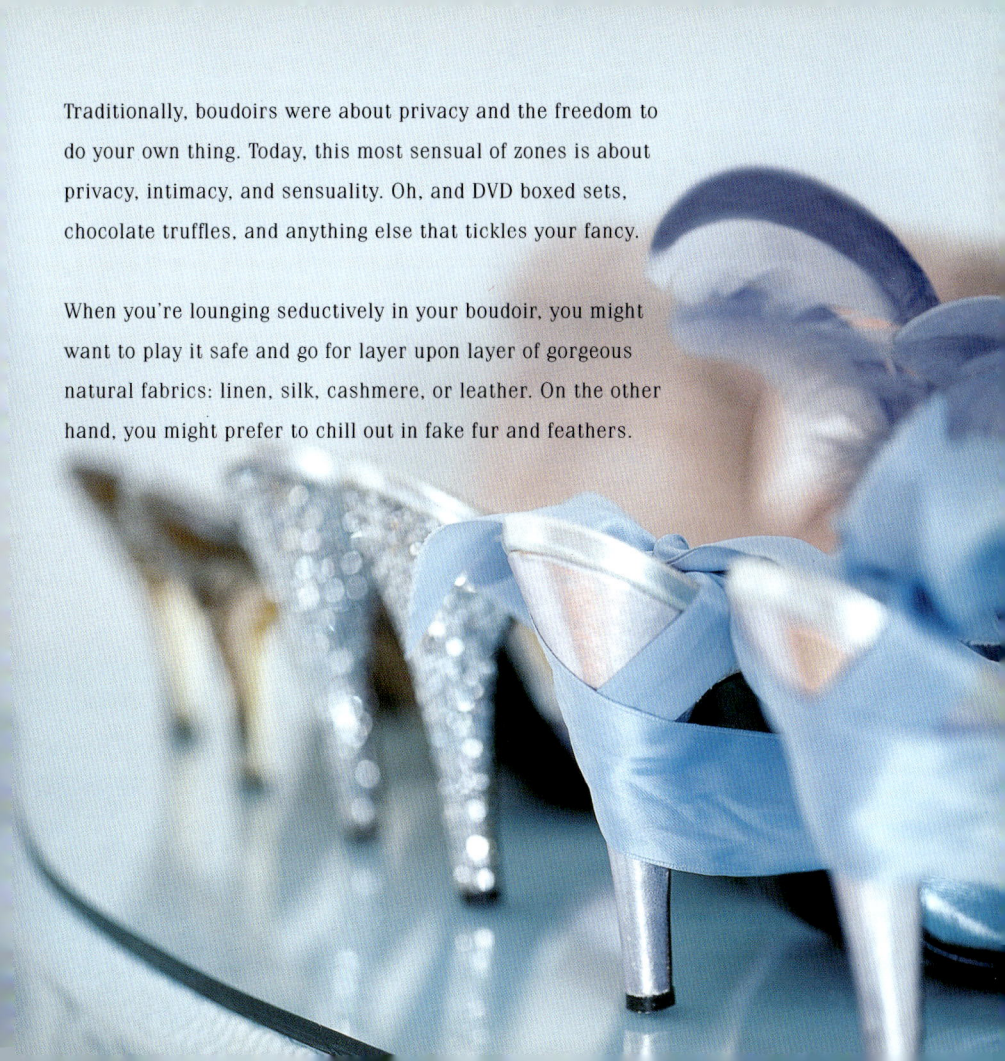

Traditionally, boudoirs were about privacy and the freedom to do your own thing. Today, this most sensual of zones is about privacy, intimacy, and sensuality. Oh, and DVD boxed sets, chocolate truffles, and anything else that tickles your fancy.

When you're lounging seductively in your boudoir, you might want to play it safe and go for layer upon layer of gorgeous natural fabrics: linen, silk, cashmere, or leather. On the other hand, you might prefer to chill out in fake fur and feathers.

> *"Licence my roving hands, and let them go, Before, behind, between, above, below."*
>
> FROM *TO HIS MISTRESS GOING TO BED* BY JOHN DONNE (1573–1631)

You may feel playful and venture into exclusive erotic boutiques (or at least pay a discreet visit to their websites) and toy with the idea of buying a pink mousseline peekaboo teddy and mirroring the bedroom ceiling. OK, so the reality may fall short of the fantasy, but it's definitely worth a look!

Heels at home are heaven sent. There's no teetering along dirty sidewalks or getting your heel stuck in a manhole cover. In the boudoir, what's called for are stilettos that are easy to kick off seductively as you curl up. Spike-heeled mules fit the bill perfectly—consider those fashioned from softest pink marabou feathers, satin, and ribbons. Lounging in your boudoir is all about confidence, femininity, and seduction. (Alternatively, you could always just settle down with a book and have a good go at those chocolate truffles…)

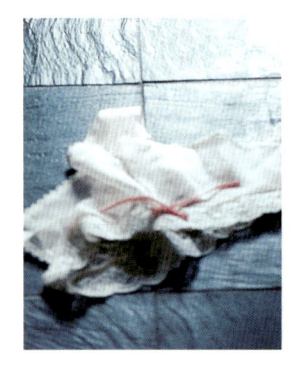

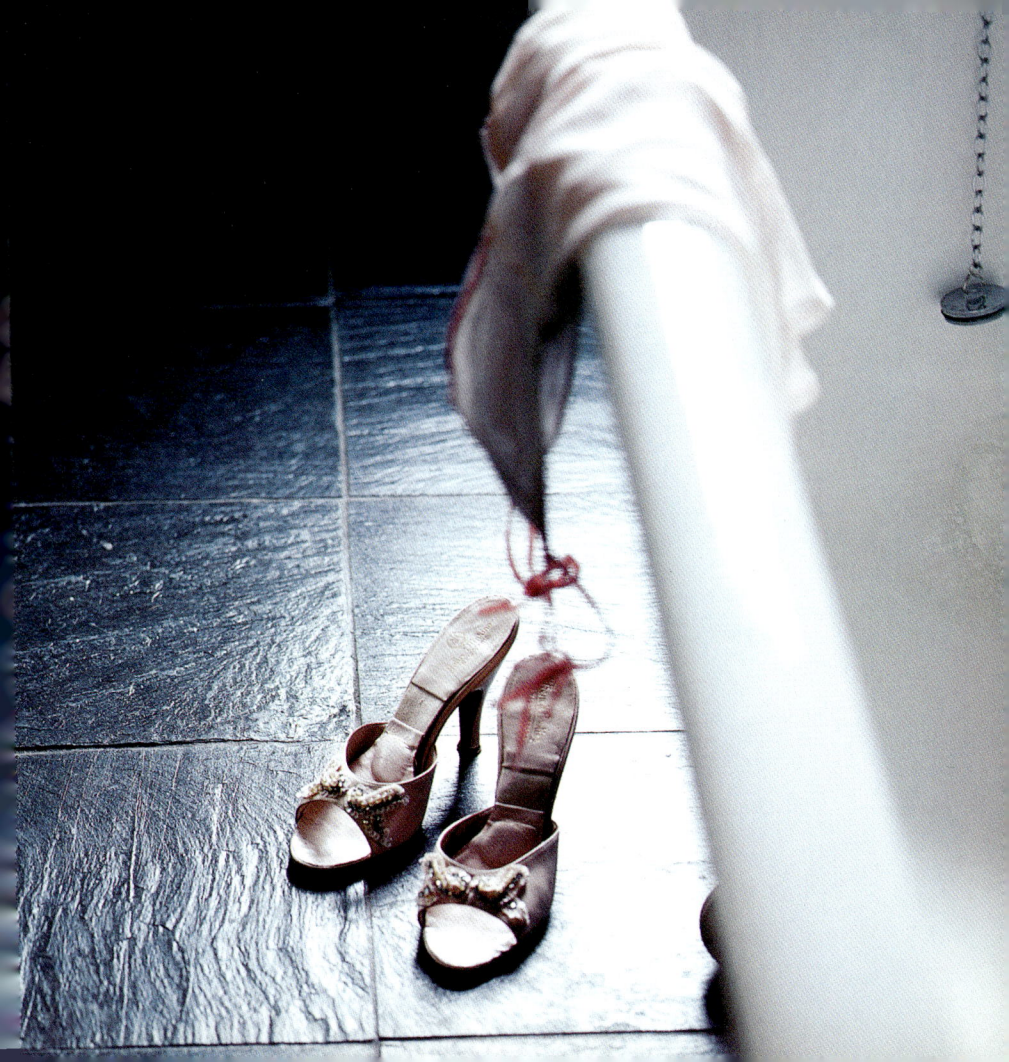

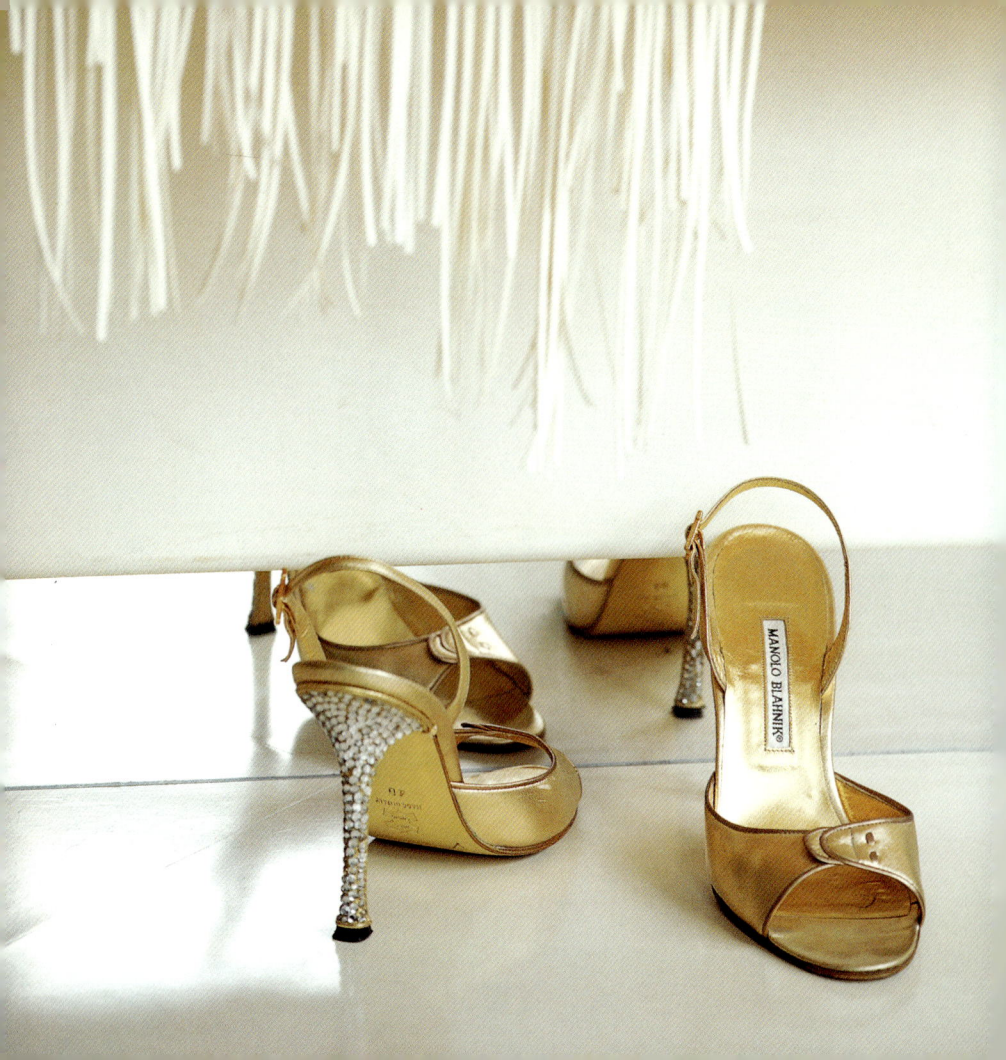

SPECIAL OCCASIONS

kick up your heels

> "Mount on French heels when you go to a ball, 'Tis the fashion to totter and show you can fall."
>
> 18TH-CENTURY SATIRICAL POEM

Whether or not you've integrated needle heels into your everyday life, when there's a special occasion it's time to up the ante. The bold will start with a divine pair of stilettos and build their outfit around them. This approach is similar to those lucky people with vision who will fall in love with one painting, vase, or lamp, then use that piece as their inspiration for a whole interior.

Historically, very special stilettos have been commissioned and worn for very special occasions. Roger Vivier created a pair of heels for Queen Elizabeth II to wear on her coronation. In curving strands of gold leather, the heels were encrusted with real garnets.

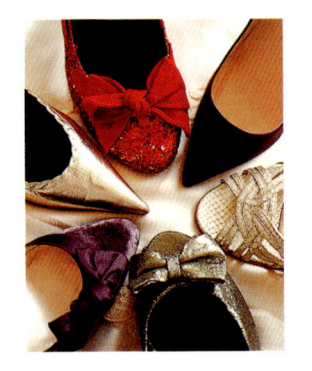

Today, the red carpet wouldn't be the same without film stars attempting to stride across the deep pile on pin-sharp five-inch designer heels. Nor, for that matter, would a wedding feel quite right without a legion of female guests wobbling across the church's parking lot or click-clacking down the aisle with verve to take their seat.

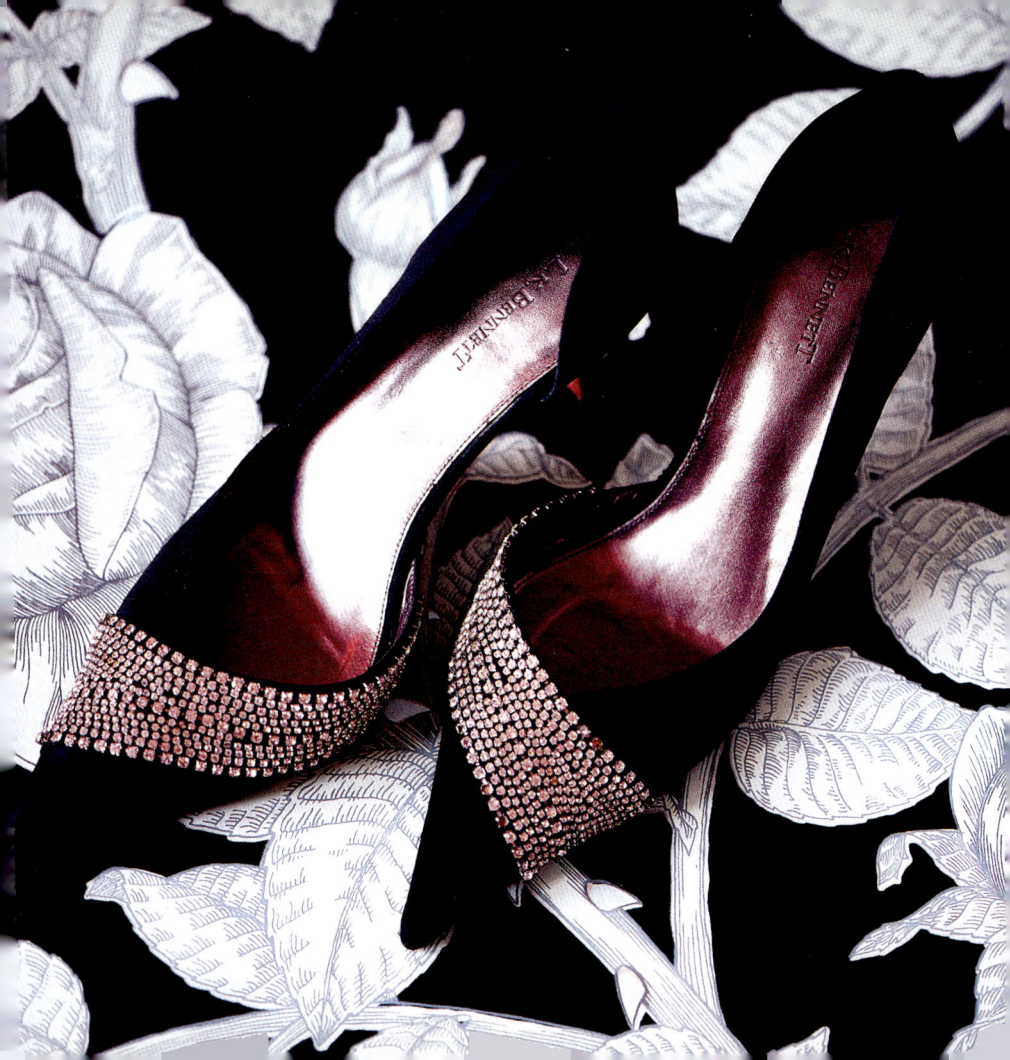

*"Down the long and silent street
The dawn, with silver-sandaled feet
Crept like a frightened girl."*

FROM *THE HARLOT'S HOUSE*
BY OSCAR WILDE (1854–1900)

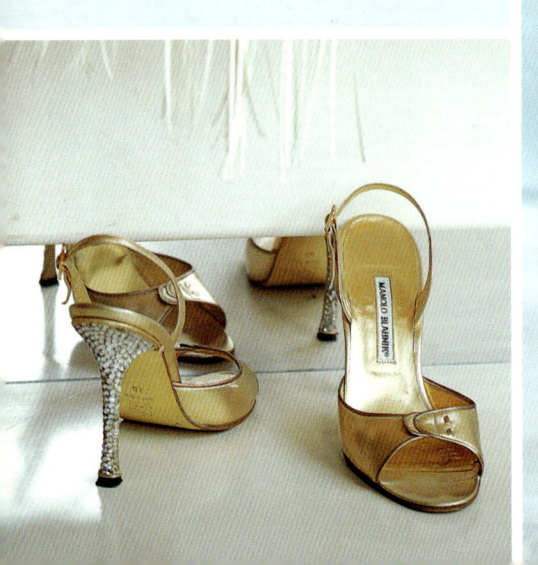

Sadly, not many of us can afford to hire a designer to create a custom-made pair of stilettos for us, but don't dismay—next time you're going shoe shopping, just make a special event out of the whole experience.

If possible, set aside a whole day for the shoe search. And make sure you really do your research. Think about where you are heading, and build in plenty of treats along the way. By treats, we're talking anything from a pomegranate martini in a hip hotel bar to a dainty afternoon tea with scones and sandwiches, or whatever other treats might tickle your fancy.

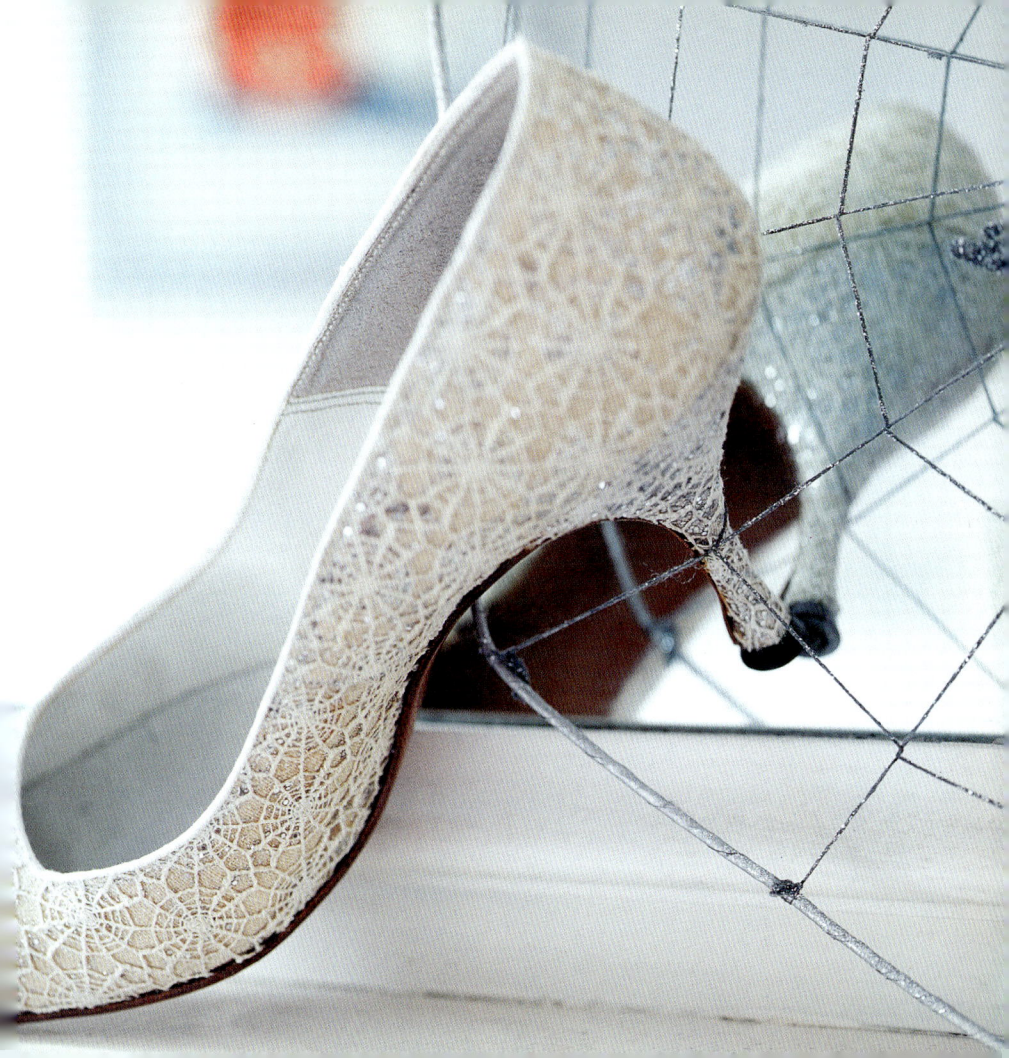

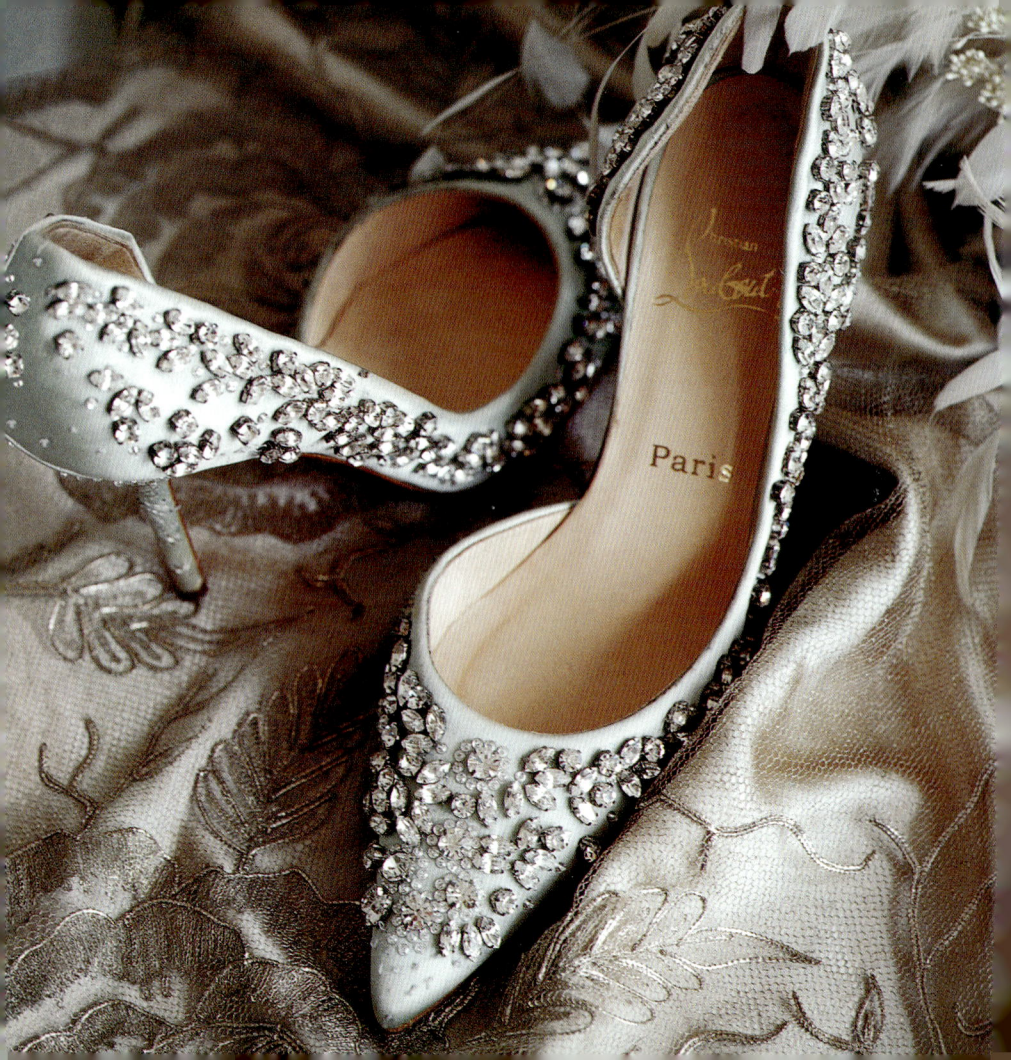

> *"So you'll measure me, please, for shoes—and shoes That will wear for years and years; And you'll make me a pair that shall fit me well, Of leather and thread, and—tears."*
>
> FROM *THE ROMANCE OF THE SHOE* (1922) BY THOMAS WRIGHT (DATES UNKNOWN)

The point is that you must enjoy every single minute of the day of purchase. Similarly, when your shoes are about to embark upon their very first outing, make sure you catch them on camera, just as you would a new baby. These shoes are going to have a great time in life!

It goes without saying that special occasions should always necessitate a special toe-grooming session. Book a pedicure for a day or two before the big event. On the day itself, allow yourself plenty of time to get ready. We don't want you shoving your feet into your shoes at the last minute without appreciating every second of the experience.

What's called for here is a languorous and appreciative preparatory ritual. Once you're perfectly coiffed and fully made up, have slipped into your best clothes, and—last but not least—your precious new shoes are on, a glass of champagne, sipped slowly before you leave, is always welcome (mind you, gulping a glass down in two seconds flat also works wonders!).

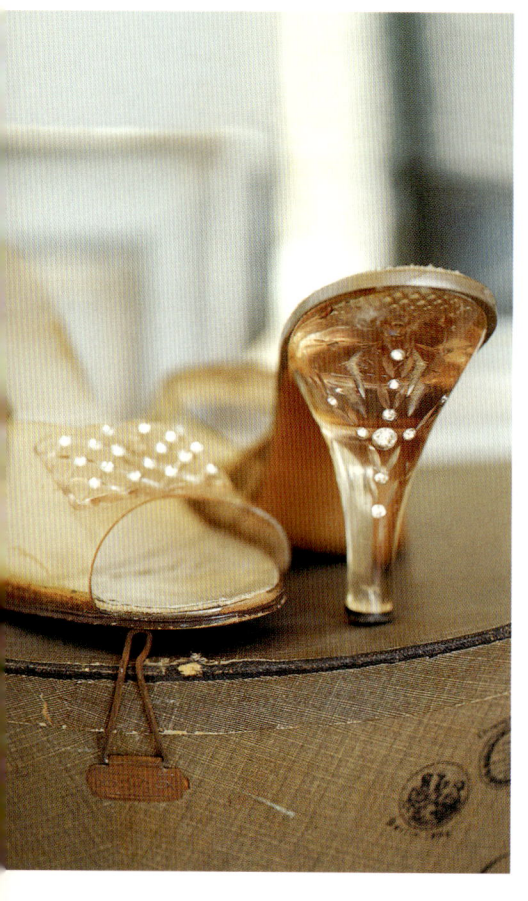

walking on air

In *Gentlemen Prefer Blondes*, when Jane Russell announces that her feet are killing her, Marilyn Monroe reminds her that a lady should *never* say that her feet hurt. Today a lady never needs to, thanks to the wonders of modern technology in the form of gel-cushioned insoles.

Now if you are lucky enough to buy Manolos, due to their legendary comfort you won't be needing any of this gel-cushion nonsense. But for the rest of us they are a nifty invention and well worth a try. After all, you could have a red-carpet sashay, a down-the-aisle glide, and an all-guns-blazing tango to deal with. And that's all before the real dancing starts. So if you plan to go the distance, it's good to do it in comfort. Well, less discomfort, at least…

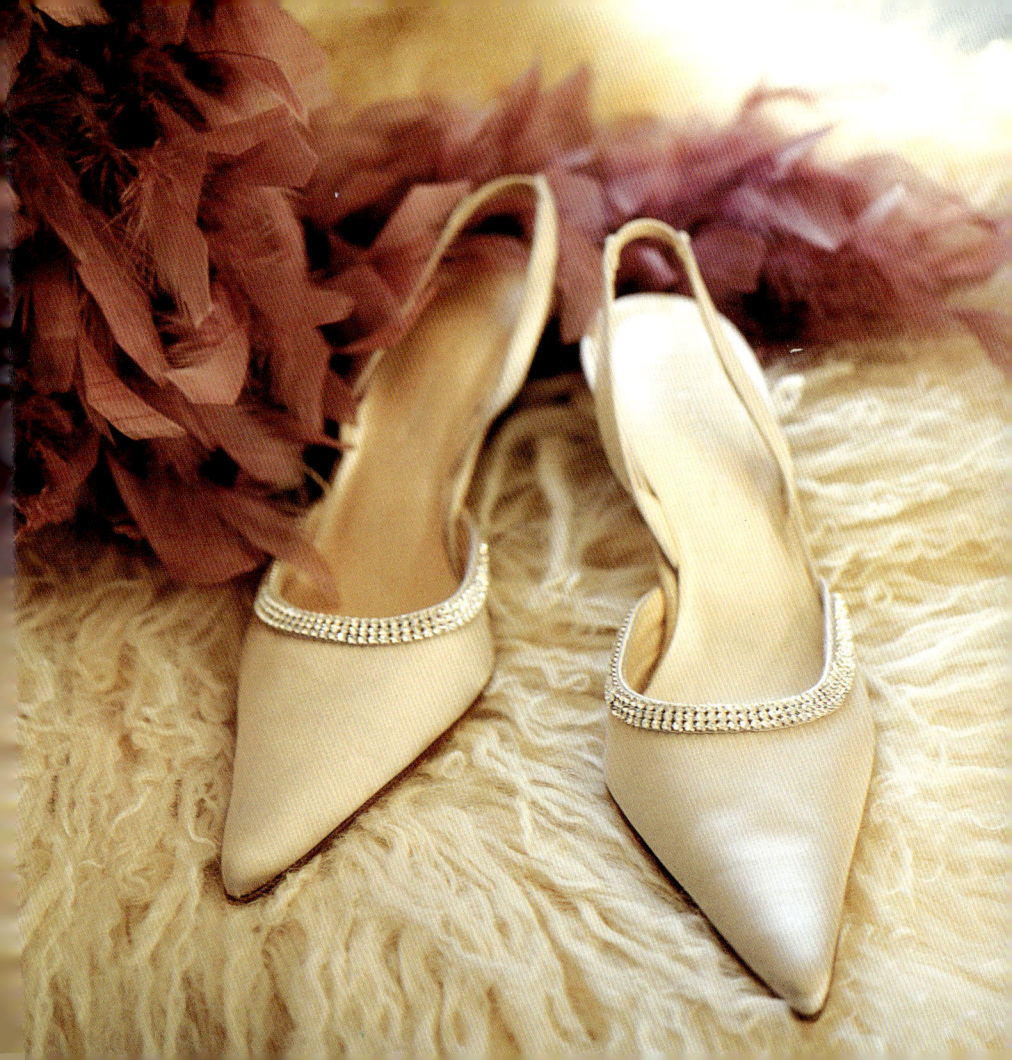

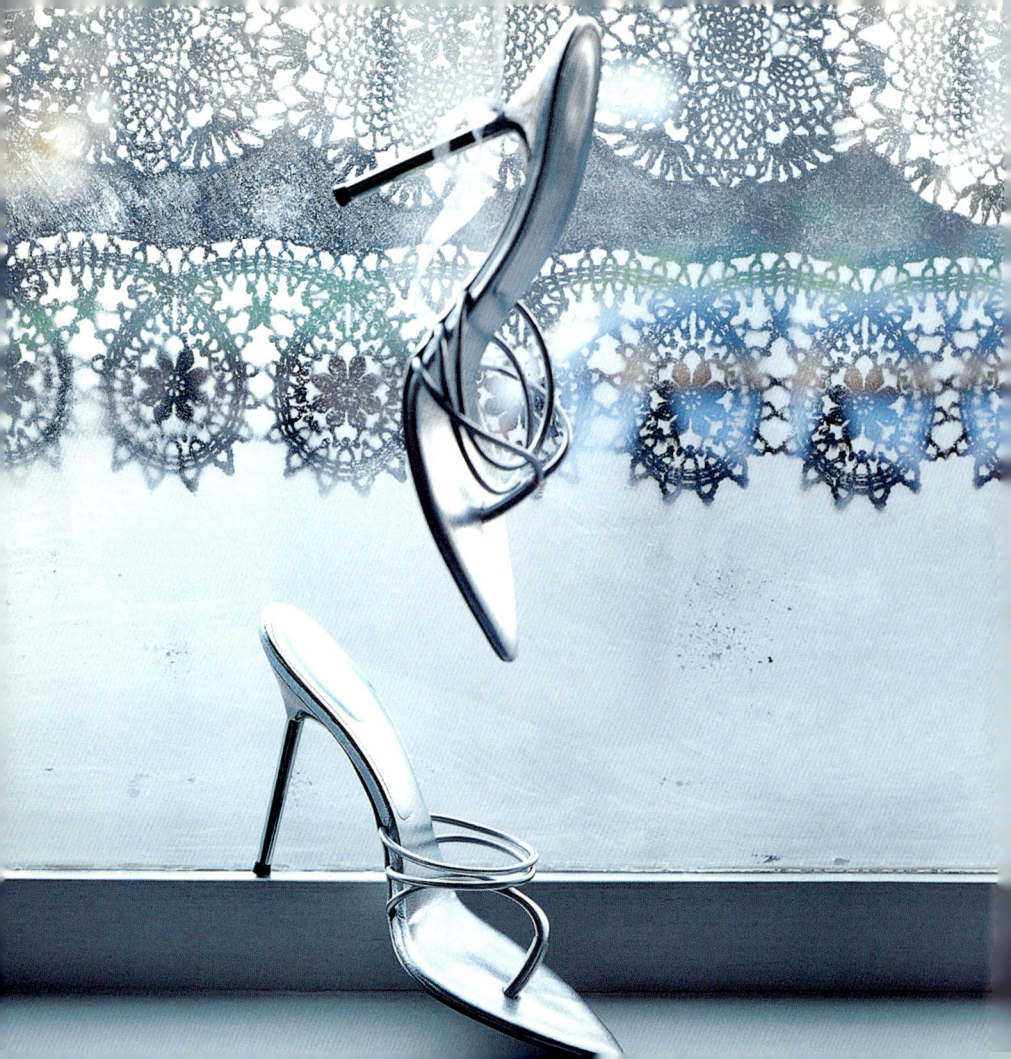

how to walk in heels

1. Do some exercises. If you did ballet, then a few toe-flexing exercises will fit the bill nicely. What's key is to get your feet used to the big flex.
2. Practise first wearing high shoes with chunkier heels.
3. It goes without saying that, for stilettos, only perfectly pedicured feet will do. The next time you have a professional pedicure, pay attention to what goes on. Invest in the equipment and set up your own mini home spa.
4. For your first outing, bare feet (as opposed to stockinged) are a good idea, as they offer more grip.
5. On the shoes go. Up, up, and away! If you do yoga, adopt Tadasana, or mountain pose. If you don't, then find your center of gravity.
6. Look in the mirror. Shoulders back. Smile! Think relaxed, graceful thoughts.
7. Take your first few steps. Unlike walking in flats, where the form is heel, ball, toe, in stilettos your feet should land flat on the floor.
8. Tackling stairs: going up, land on the ball of your foot. Going down, side step, toes pointing in the same direction.
9. It's time to get out and about. Much has been said about stilettos and taxis, and it's all true. You won't go far on five-inch heels, but what's important is that those short "car to bar" journeys look really smooth.
10. Once you become an expert, there's no excuse. None of this "heels are for high days and holidays" nonsense. Every day can be a high day. So don't drag your heels—be bold, smile, and flex those arches.

business credits

BIBA LIVES
Stand number G014–22
Alfie's Antique Market
13–25 Church Street
London NW8 8DT
+44 20 7258 7999
www.bibalives.com

CHRISTIAN LOUBOUTIN
23 Motcomb Street
London SW1X 8LB
+44 20 7245 6510

GIL CARVALHO
+44 20 7262 2658
www.gilcarvalho.com

KURT GEIGER
+44 845 257 2571
www.kurtgeiger.com

LAURA BROOKS
+44 7748 187264
By appointment.
laurabrooks@laurabrooks.co.uk

LULU GUINNESS
+44 20 7823 4828
www.luluguinness.com

MAISONETTE
79 Chamberlayne Road
London NW10 3ND
+44 20 8964 8444
www.maisonette.uk.com

MYLA
77 Lonsdale Road
London W11 2DF
+44 8707 455003
www.myla.com

OFFICE SHOES
www.office.co.uk

RACHEL KELLY
Interactive Wallpaper
+44 20 7490 3076
www.interactivewallpaper.co.uk

THE GIRL CAN'T HELP IT
Stand number G080–100
Alfie's Antique Market
13–25 Church Street
London NW8 8DT
+44 20 7724 8984
www.thegirlcanthelpit.com

TIN TIN COLLECTABLES
Stand number G038–42
Alfie's Antique Market
13–25 Church Street
London NW8 8DT
+44 20 7258 1305
www.tintincollectables.com

V V ROULEAUX
6 Marylebone High Street
London W1U 4NJ
+44 20 7224 5179
www.vvrouleaux.com

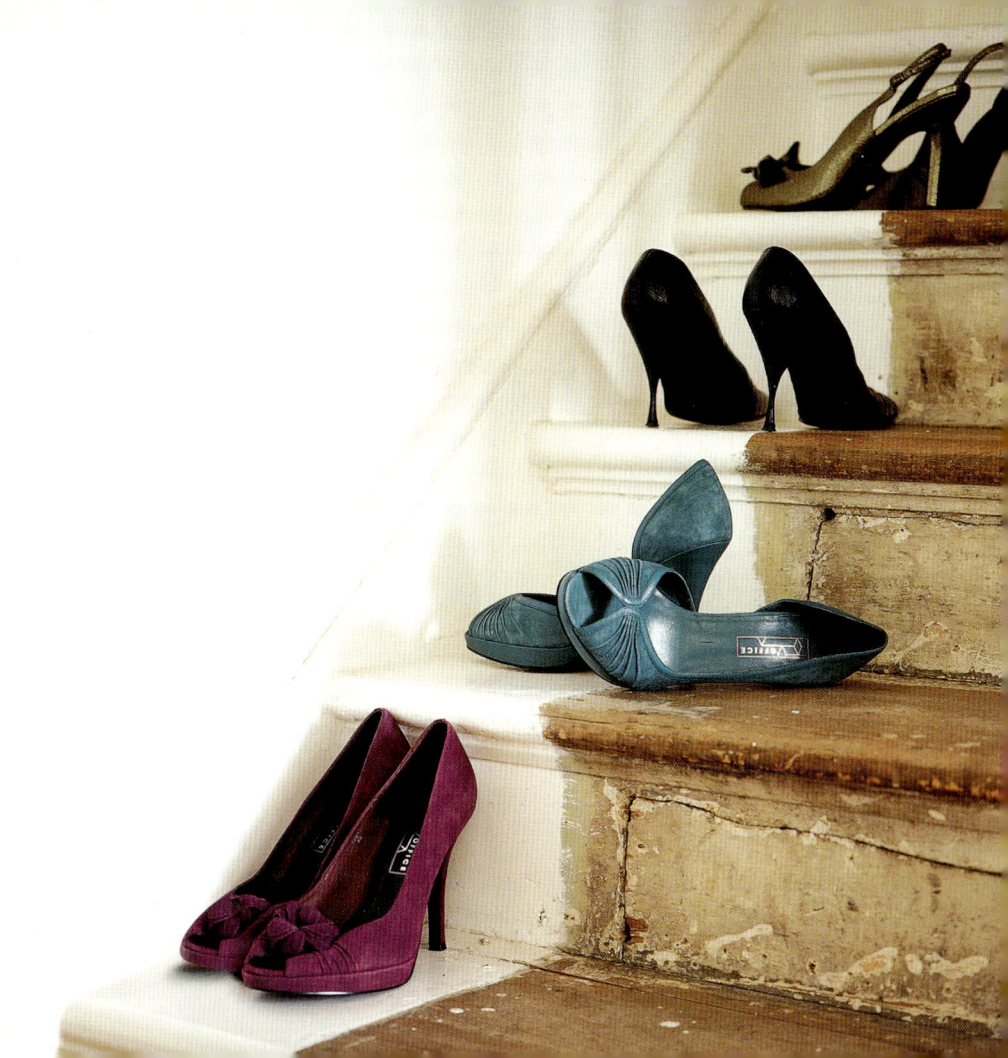

picture credits

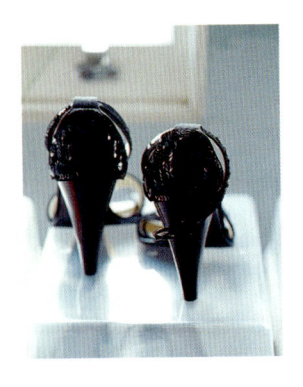

All photography by Sandra Lane.
Key: a=above, b=below, r=right,
l=left, c=center.

De Roemer
42 Casselden Road
London NW10 8QR
tel: + 44 20 8965 1602
fax: + 44 20 8961 8737
www.deroemer.com
Pages 26–27, 42, 53, 59, 64a

Julia Clancey
www.juliaclancey.com
Pages 4c inset, 31, 40–41, 46–47, 55

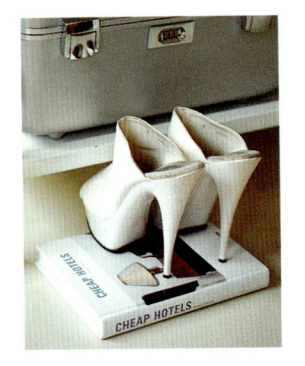

acknowledgments

Thank you Natasha, for giving me my first Jimmy Choo experience. And thank you Sarah for many shoe stories—and inspiration from your poem "Wearing DMs in Spain." And a very big thank you to Michael Keet, the most wonderful reflexologist.

The publishers would like to thank all those who allowed us to photograph in their homes for this book, including special thanks to fashion and jewelry designer Julia Clancey, Ros Fairman, and Justin Packshaw and Tamsin De Roemer.

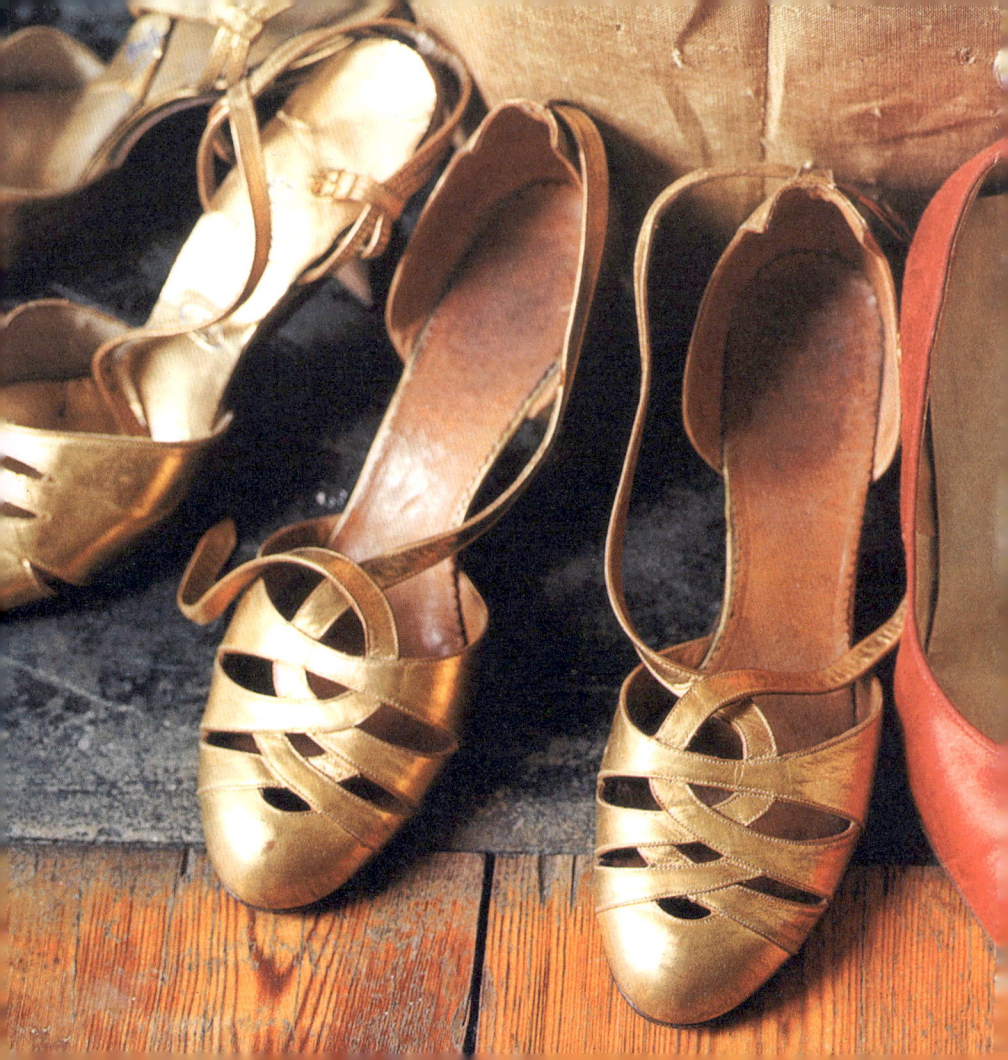